Parasites and Western Man

Parasites and Western Man

EDITED BY

R. J. Donaldson

Director of Studies
Centre for Extension Training
in Community Medicine
London School of Hygiene and
Tropical Medicine

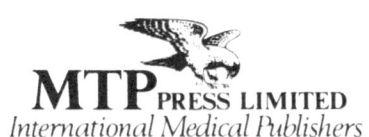

MTPPRESS LIMITED
International Medical Publishers

Published by
MTP Press Limited
Falcon House
Lancaster, England

British Library Cataloguing in Publication Data

Parasites and Western Man
1. Medical parasitology
I. Donaldson, Raymond Joseph
616.9′6′0091722   RC119

ISBN-13: 978-94-011-6196-1   e-ISBN-13: 978-94-011-6194-7
DOI: 10.1007/ 978-94-011-6194-7

Text set in 11/12pt Photon Times

Contents

List of Contributors

R. E. Church
Consultant Dermatologist
The Rupert Hallam Department of Dermatology
The Hallamshire Hospital
Sheffield

R. J. Donaldson
Director of Studies
Centre for Extension Training in Community Medicine
London School of Hygiene and Tropical Medicine
London

T. E. Gibson
Head
Department of Parasitology
Central Veterinary Laboratory
Ministry of Agriculture, Fisheries and Food
Weybridge

H. M. Gilles
Alfred Jones and Warrington Yorke Professor of Tropical Medicine
Liverpool School of Tropical Medicine
Liverpool University
Liverpool

D. E. Jacobs
Senior Lecturer
Department of Microbiology and Parasitology
The Royal Veterinary College
London

J. W. Maunder
Lecturer
Department of Entomology
London School of Hygiene and Tropical Medicine
London

R. Muller
Senior Lecturer
Department of Medical Helminthology
London School of Hygiene and Tropical Medicine
London

G. S. Nelson
William Julien Courtauld Professor of Medical Helminthology
London School of Hygiene and Tropical Medicine
London

D. R. Seaton
Clinical Lecturer
Department of Tropical Medicine
Liverpool School of Tropical Medicine
Liverpool University
Liverpool

Preface

The purpose of this book is to provide a concise account of those parasites which affect man in developed countries. Other textbooks relate mainly to the tropics and subtropics where parasites by comparison are more common. It is widely believed that this difference in prevalence between tropical and temperate countries is due to differences in climatic conditions alone. Whilst it is true that certain vectors can only act as transmitters of disease under climatic conditions found in the tropics, there are many other instances where climate *per se* is not a decisive factor. More often parasitic disease is related to the poor standards of hygiene, sanitation and nutrition, which characterize many of these tropical and subtropical areas. The advent of more international travel has added a new dimension to the study of parasites, with the appearance of rare and exotic parasitic infections in the West.

This book encompasses the entire field of parasites in developed countries with a brief reference to other parts of the world whenever appropriate for the sake of completeness.

Each chapter provides basic information as well as recent advances and current thinking. Thus the book will serve as an excellent, comprehensive introduction to those taking up a specialized interest in the subject, as well as those who may wish to obtain general information but are not actively working in the field. Although it is primarily written from a medical and veterinary standpoint, it provides valuable material for other disciplines.

The individual chapters have been contributed by people who practise and have been involved in research in the fields about which they write. They are all experienced teachers of students and graduates of different disciplines. Nearly all the authors have provided extensive reference lists so that a reader can explore a particular aspect of a topic in greater depth. Emphasis throughout the book is placed on prevention.

The currently accepted treatment is described for each of the conditions discussed and it is also indicated where treatment is unnecessary. The first chapter examines in a general way the host–parasite relationship—often an uneasy relationship possibly because man has been on this planet for so short a period in the evolutionary time-scale. It is thus important to keep in perspective the need for intervention to avoid disrupting this fragile balance. There are separate chapters on insect parasites, nematodes, cestodes and trematodes, and protozoa. A detailed account of scabies is included in the chapter on mites and ticks. Infestation by head lice, which appears to be more prevalent in Western societies, is examined in detail in a separate chapter. The final contributions from my veterinary colleagues give a balanced viewpoint of the risks to man from his pets and domestic animals.

I am most grateful to the chapter writers for their help. During the final stages of the preparation of this text, I gladly acknowledge the generous help given to me by Jean Coyle, Liam Donaldson, MB, MSc, FRCS (Ed), Nicola Spencer, BSc and Peter Waters, MA. I was fortunate in having a helpful, friendly and cooperative publisher who exhibited infinite patience with the problems that arose from producing this multi-author book.

Dr R J Donaldson, OBE
Director of Studies
Centre for Extension Training in Community Medicine
Department of Community Medicine
London School of Hygiene and Tropical Medicine

1
The Parasite and the Host

G. S. NELSON

INTRODUCTION

The phenomenon of parasitism occurs amongst all groups of infective agents whether they are viruses, bacteria, fungi, protozoa, helminths or arthropods. The main concern of this book is with the protozoa, helminths and arthropods, parasites that are still of public health importance in economically advanced societies. Our main concern is with the parasites which are naturally transmitted in advanced countries. It is not generally realized that there are several parasitic organisms which maintain themselves in these countries with very high prevalence rates; in fact we are all infected at some time in our lives with at least one type of parasite and many people even in the most advanced societies have the ciliated *Trichomonas* in their genital tracts, the intracellular parasite *Toxoplasma* in their reticulo-endothelial system, the pinworm *Enterobius* in their bowel, and the wingless insect *Demodex* under their skin. Most people are completely unaware that they are infected and even when they have symptoms the diagnosis is seldom made. Usually they are harmless commensals and as we will see later in this chapter they may even be beneficial symbionts stimulating our immune system so that we reject more pathogenic organisms.

Most of the parasites that are naturally transmitted in advanced societies are more prevalent in underdeveloped tropical regions of the world, but the increase in world travel for pleasure or for business and the mass movements of immigrants and emigrants means that some of the parasites that were becoming rare in the developed world are being reintroduced into areas where transmission can occur. For example there is a danger of the reintroduction of malaria, hookworms and filariasis into the warmer regions of Europe and North America where these infections have almost been eliminated; these parasites require special vigilance by the public health authorities. Western man is particularly at risk of developing exotic infections. He has lost his

1

acquired immunity and when he returns from a visit to the tropics his infection may go unrecognized.

THE PARASITE–HOST RELATIONSHIP

The term parasitism implies that the organism lives at the expense of the host but this is too narrow a concept; the same organisms can at different times be harmful, innocuous or beneficial depending on the site they inhabit and the stimulus they produce. If two creatures live in close association with one another, one gaining benefit, the other suffering no harm, this is commensalism, the classical example being the sucker fish on the belly of the shark. Where both gain benefit from the association this is symbiosis, for example herbivorous animals require protozoa in their guts to help with digestion and we know from the occasional disastrous effects of antibiotics that man requires a complex bacterial fauna in his gut to prevent the overgrowth of fungi. Symbiosis and mutualism are synonymous and sometimes the terms can be extended to embrace man's relationship with his domestic animals and pets, the domestic cat repaying his mistress by catching rats and mice, but the relationship is not always beneficial. The cat harbours a variety of parasites that can infect man and the same is even more true of the dog. The relationship between the dog and its master can be described as symbiotic in the case of the watchdog, the sheepdog, the hunting dog and even the lapdog which brings comfort and companionship to its owner but dogs share more than 50 infective organisms with man and the relationship is not always to the mutual advantage of man and his 'best friend'.

PATHOGENICITY

In terms of their pathogenicity the protozoa have much in common with bacteria and viruses in that they are capable of multiplying within the host and a single exposure can result in heavy infection. This is not the case with most of the helminths where there is no multiplication in man and where the severity of the disease is proportional to the worm load and this in turn depends on the intensity of transmission. The more severe manifestations of the disease usually depend on the accumulation of parasites from repeated exposure but with the protozoa and helminths, as with other organisms, it is the strain of the parasite and the susceptibility of the host which determines the severity of the disease.

Most pathological reactions are determined either by an intrinsic genetic resistance or susceptibility to infection or by an acquired resistance. For example it has been known for many years that negroes in West Africa were not infected with *Plasmodium vivax* and that negroes in North America could not be infected with this parasite when it was used for pyrotherapy in cerebral syphilis. It has now been shown that this particular malarial parasite fails to infect negroes because their red cells are deficient in the appropriate surface receptors. Many negroes are also less susceptible to heavy infections with the malignant tertian parasite *P. falciparum* than Caucasians, but in this case a different mechanism is involved and the protection only occurs in those carrying the sickle cell trait.

Variability in the parasites may be of even greater significance than host factors in determining the outcome of parasitic infections. For example there are several forms of *Echinococcus granulosus* producing hydatid cysts in animals and although they are morphologically similar they show considerable host specificity. The common *E. granulosus* of sheep and dogs is infective to man, thus hydatid disease occurs in the western areas of the United Kingdom where this parasite is prevalent. However in the eastern counties of England horses and hunting dogs are much more heavily infected with *Echinococcus* and yet there is no hydatid disease in man. It has been shown that this strain of the parasite has a more restricted host range and epidemiological evidence suggests that man is unlikely to become infected. Another parasite showing variability is *Trichinella spiralis*, one of the most primitive worms with a cosmopolitan distribution. Until quite recently it was thought that the hosts *par excellence* for this parasite were rats and domestic pigs but studies in Africa, the USSR and Canada have shown that the real reservoirs of this parasite are cannibalistic or carrion-feeding carnivores and that some wild strains, e.g. from the Arctic regions, southern Europe and Africa, are not infective to rats and pigs. These differences in infectivity or host susceptibility have a profound influence on the epidemiology of parasitic disease[1].

Helminthologists have been slow to recognize that morphological identity is no guarantee of identical behaviour; on the other hand protozoologists have always been conscious of the problem of intraspecific variations in determining the epidemiology of protozoological infections but only recently have they discovered means of separating many of the different forms of trypanosomes, leishmania and entamoebae other than by the character of the disease they produced. The development of isoenzyme mapping is superseding many of the less reliable biological and immunological techniques for distinguishing morphologically identical protozoa with very different pathogenic and epidemiological properties[2].

Parasites, with their bizarre pathology, often cause confusion in diagnosis, especially in countries where they are uncommon. For example, malaria parasites destroy the red blood cells thus producing a haemolytic anaemia, but they also block capillaries in the brain and in some cases coma develops rapidly and the patient then dies because of failure to make a diagnosis. The same is true of African trypanosomiasis; the classical sleeping sickness is easily recognized in the endemic areas but in returning travellers the encephalitis with chronic headache and strange mental symptoms will often not be diagnosed, particularly if the physician is unaware that the patient has travelled in Africa. South American trypanosomiasis has an even more complex pathology, with the parasite multiplying in the heart muscle and nervous tissues of the gut, the resulting heart failure and gross enlargement of the oesophagus or colon causing diagnostic confusion. Many of the intestinal amoebae are harmless commensals and some are probably beneficial symbionts, but the occasional virulent forms of *Entamoeba hystolytica* can cause tissue necrosis with deep ulcers of the bowel or ectopic abscesses in the liver, whilst the usually harmless *Naegleria* has caused brain abscesses and an allergic reaction to this organism is now thought to be responsible for pneumonitis caused by humidifiers in factories[3]. The intestinal ciliate *Giardia lamblia*, which is a relatively harmless parasite in most parts of the world, has gained notoriety in recent years as a cause of persistent travellers' diarrhoea and the malabsorption syndrome which is frequently seen in tourists returning to the United States and Europe from the USSR and especially in 'overlanders' returning from Nepal and India. These tiny protozoa are present in enormous numbers attached to the villi of the small intestine but travellers' diarrhoea and the accompanying malabsorption syndrome is more liable to be attributed to a viral or bacterial infection and the parasitic aetiology remains unrecognized.

The wasting child or the thin animal is often said to have worms on the assumption that intestinal parasites deny man a considerable proportion of his food. This is very rarely true even with very heavy worm loads. The pathogenesis is usually more subtle and helminths like protozoa can cause considerable diagnostic confusion. In Finland whole communities are infected with the fish tapeworm *Diphyllobothrium latum* (an enormous worm often several metres long) but very few people are even conscious of the infection. This is usually diagnosed by a haematologist who recognizes the pernicious anaemia caused by the worm's ability to absorb vitamin B_{12} into its cuticle. The common *Ascaris* roundworms, although present in large numbers, rarely cause trouble except by the initial wandering of the larvae through the lungs, producing Loeffler's syndrome with pneumonitis and a high eosinophilia, or in the later stage by the adult worms obstructing the bowel or the bile ducts. Hookworms may be present in very large numbers with as many as 1000 worms in the small intestine with little in the way of symptoms other than abdominal discomfort which might be misdiagnosed as peptic ulcer. The characteristic hookworm anaemia only develops when the iron stores have been depleted and this takes many months in people with a deficient intake of iron and may never occur in people on a good diet who remain in positive iron balance.

Many of the pathological changes in helminth infections are caused by inflammation or immunopathological reactions with eosinophilia as a characteristic accompaniment. The reaction may be most severe when the parasites are poorly adapted to man and when they are being rejected or encapsulated. For example the dog parasite *Toxocara* is usually rejected without symptoms but it can produce severe lesions in eyes of children which may be misdiagnosed as neuroblastomas or non-specific granulomas. Because the parasite fails to reach maturity in man there are no eggs in the faeces and serological tests are necessary to establish a diagnosis. This is the case with many abortive zoonoses where man is an abnormal host of parasites of animals. Another example is cercarial dermatitis which results from infection with bird schistosomes. This caused some confusion in diagnosis when it occurred amongst competitors at an international water-ski-ing championship in England[4]. Again indirect methods of diagnosis were necessary. Herring-worm disease and other helminthomas of the bowel, such as those caused by oesophagostomes of monkeys, often result in unnecessary major surgery, the eosinophilic granulomas caused by these parasites being mistaken for tumours.

Heavy infections with the more pathogenic helminths are rarely seen outside the endemic areas but with the increasing affluence of the less developed countries, more and more patients are seeking treatment in Europe and North America and patients with advanced pathology of diseases such as schistosomiasis or filariasis are no longer a rarity in our hospitals.

IN PERSPECTIVE

One of the tragic problems of parasitic diseases and particularly helminth infection is that patients become obsessed with a repugnance which creates severe psychotic disturbances. This occurs not only with the large relatively harmless tapeworms and roundworms but with the much more prevalent threadworms which, apart from psychological problems, rarely produce anything more severe than occasional pruritus. There is a need for greater knowledge and greater awareness of parasites not only by medical and public health workers but by the general public. We must be careful not to exaggerate the problems.

Education may already have gone too far in overemphasizing the danger of lice and fleas. The diseases they transmit, typhus and plague, are no longer a threat to our urban societies and although it is aesthetically desirable and prophylactically wise to eliminate these pests it is unfortunate if those who are lousy with harmless head lice or those who are fleabitten by harmless dog fleas are made neurotic by listening to too much exaggerated propaganda.

We must also be aware of the gross exaggeration and almost terrifying campaigns that have been mounted to make the population aware of the dangers of zoonotic diseases such as rabies and toxocariasis. These campaigns have caused untold misery to many old people who have deep emotional relationships with their pets and who now feel conscience stricken because they are keeping cats and dogs which they are told are a public health menace. Rabies is an extremely rare human disease even in areas where the organism is highly prevalent in wild animal reservoirs such as the fox in Europe or the vampire bat in South America. Toxocariasis is similarly prevalent in wild carnivores and domestic dogs and serological tests suggest that man is commonly infected with the developing larvae, but it is a rare disease which only excites the academic physician or the over-conscientious environmental sanitation expert and it is not a public health problem of any significance.

ZOONOSES

Man acquires many of his parasites from animals and, like most of the major infectious diseases in the world, they are zoonoses with animals as the true maintenance hosts of the organisms in nature. The term zoonosis is useful in focusing attention on the ways in which animal infections are transmitted to man. It is a dynamic concept implying the to and fro movement of infection between different hosts, some which are well adapted, carrying inapparent infections without diseases, others producing more obvious pathology and clinically recognizable disease. A joint committee of the World Health Organization and the Food and Agricultural Organization defined the zoonoses as 'those diseases and infections naturally transmitted between man and other vertebrates'. It is an old concept enshrined in the Mosaic law and in the Koran. In Deuteronomy Chapter 14 Verse 8 Moses says: 'And the swine it is unclean unto you—ye shall not eat of their flesh nor touch their dead carcases', and Verse 21: 'Ye shall not eat anything that dieth of itself.'

In the days of Moses, trichinosis, cysticercosis and salmonellosis were all likely to be acquired from pigs. The carcasses of animals that had died could have been a sure source of anthrax. The law of Moses, which was reinforced by Mohammed, must have saved millions of Jews and Moslems from developing diseases transmitted by pigs or from animals that 'die of themselves' but Moses was probably unaware of the public health significance of his doctrine (or less scrupulous than we are led to believe) because later in the same chapter of Deuteronomy he says, 'Thou shalt give it unto the stranger that is in thy gate that he may eat it or thou mayest sell it unto an alien.'

Jenner was the first medical scientist to recognize that civilized man acquires disease from animals; in his famous thesis on the cause and effect of cowpox he says, 'The deviation of man from the state in which he was placed by nature seems to have proven to him a prolific source of diseases. From the love of splendour, from the indulgence of luxury and from his fondness for amusement he has familiarized himself with a great number of animals which may not usually have been intended for his amusement. The wolf disarmed of his ferocity is now pillowed in the Lady's lap. The cat, the little tiger of our island, whose natural home is the forest is equally domesticated and caressed'. This was a prophetic statement. In 1798 when he wrote his thesis Jenner knew nothing about the life cycles and transmission of the many infections that man acquires from domestic and wild animals. Some of these are illustrated in Table 1.1 which shows examples of the different epidemiological categories of zoonoses occurring in Western societies. The division is based on the direction of transmission in relation to the true maintenance hosts of the organisms. Many of these produce obvious disease especially in the abnormal host but often zoonotic infections are either inapparent or innocuous. Benjamin Jesty, the Devonshire farmer, who preceded Jenner, was aware of this when he noticed that his milkmaids who had been infected with mildly pathogenic cowpox failed

Table 1.1   Examples of zoonoses in the United Kingdom
(See Figure 1.1 illustrating the various epidemiological categories)

CATEGORY 1   Direct to man from wild animal—maintenance host

B virus, Marburg disease	Monkey	→Man (Laboratory infection)
Ornithosis, psittacosis	Bird	→Man
Leptospirosis, salmonellosis, babesiosis	Rodent	→Man
Herring-worm disease	Seal	→Herring →Man

CATEGORY 2   To man from wild animal host via domestic animal

Louping ill	Rodent	→Sheep	→Man	
Newcastle disease	Wild bird	→Poultry	→Man	
Q fever	Rodent	→Cattle	→Man	
Tuberculosis	Badger	→Cattle	→Man	
Trichinosis	Fox	→Rodent	→Pig	→Man
Toxoplasmosis	Rodent	→Cat	→Man	

CATEGORY 3   Direct to man from domestic animal—maintenance host

Cowpox, brucellosis, anthrax, tuberculosis	Cattle	→Man
Orf, liver fluke	Sheep	→Man
Salmonella, trichinosis	Pig	→Man
Ringworm, toxocariasis, *Dipylidium caninum*, hydatid	Dog	→Man

CATEGORY 4   No host specificity—maintenance host either wild or domestic animal or man

Salmonellosis	Rodent	↔Cattle ↔Man

(Best examples of this category occur in the tropics e.g. *Schistosomiasis japonica* in SE Asia or Chagas disease in South America)

CATEGORY 5   Transmission from man to domestic animal

Influenza	Man	→Pig
Streptococcus, tuberculosis	Man	→Cow

(Also many examples of pets and animals in zoological gardens acquiring bacterial and viral infections from man e.g. chimpanzees with hepatitis, monkeys with tuberculosis)

CATEGORY 6   Transmission from man to wild animal via domestic animal

(No good examples in UK)

CATEGORY 7   Transmission from man to wild animal

(No good examples in UK; a good example in the tropics is *Schistosomia haematobium* in monkeys)

CATEGORY 8   Man and domestic animal are obligatory hosts for survival of the organism

Taenia saginata	Man	↔Cow
Taenia solium	Man	↔Pig (Probably extinct in UK)

---

to develop smallpox. This prompted him to inoculate his wife with material from a cow in the hope that she also would escape the dreaded unsightly effects of smallpox. Perhaps he was aware of the nursery rhyme:

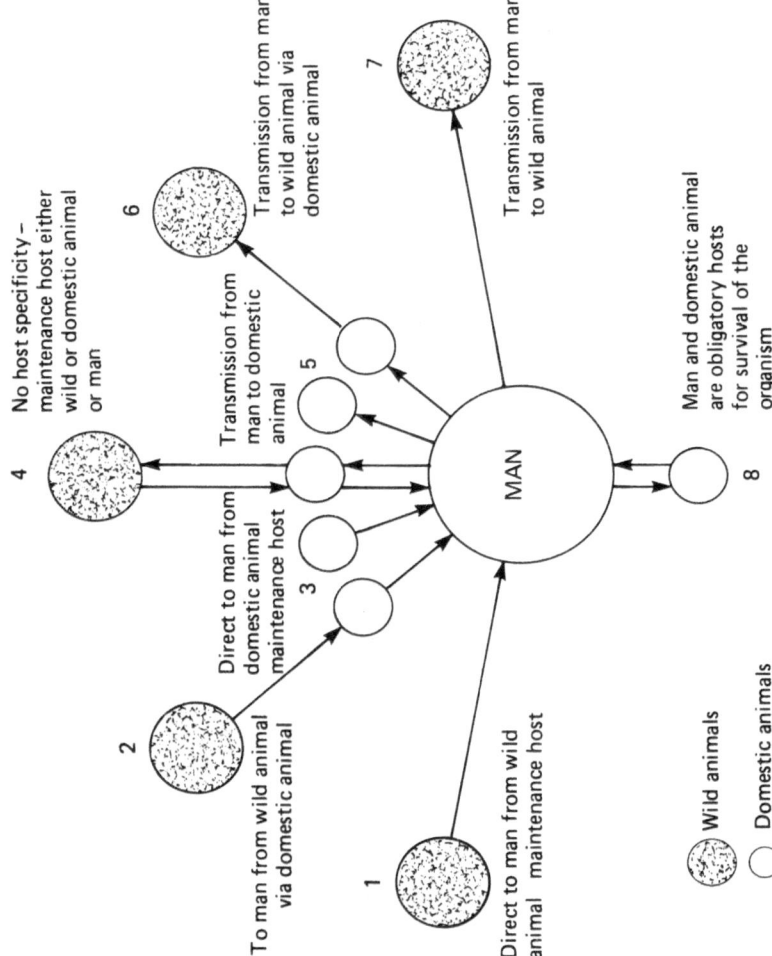

Figure 1.1   Zoonoses epidemiological categories (see Table 1.1 for examples)

'Where are you going, my pretty maid?'
'I'm going a-milking, Sir' she said.
'What is your fortune, my pretty maid?'
'My face is my fortune, Sir' she said.

Her face was her fortune because unlike her contemporaries she had escaped smallpox, because she had been previously exposed to cowpox. It was this observation which led Jenner to test the hypothesis and show by experiment that there was cross protection between cowpox and smallpox. These observations were made 200 years ago and yet we are still obsessed with organisms that produce obvious diseases and most of us are unaware of the epidemiological significance of cross protection between non-virulent and virulent organisms.

ZOOPROPHYLAXIS

This universal phenomenon may be essential for the survival of man. With most parasitic and other zoonotic infections we are concerned with the one patient in a thousand who presents with a clinically recognizable disease without wondering about the evolutionary significance of the nine hundred and ninety nine inapparent infections with the same organism. The epidemiological phenomenon of cross protection between organisms of low and high levels of pathogenicity has been referred to as zooprophylaxis which I have defined as 'the prevention or amelioration of disease in man as a result of previous exposure to heterologous infection of animal origin'. The concept can be widened to include cross protection between organisms which have escaped from their original zoonotic cycle and which are now maintained in man, for example the non-venereal treponema of yaws, which before the days of penicillin affected most of the people in the tropics and gave a high level of cross-protection against the more virulent syphilis. Also there is good epidemiological and experimental evidence of cross protection between different species of mycobacteria with inapparent infection with tuberculosis giving cross protection against leprosy.

Before we immediately condemn the parasites and try to eliminate them we need to know far more about their possible beneficial effect. For example one of the commonest infections, but at the same time rarest diseases, in the developed world is toxoplasmosis. Vast tomes have been written about the congenital malformations and eye lesions produced by this parasite. Is it possible that these misfortunes are the price we pay for the stimulus that this organism gives the cell-mediated immune response of millions of people who acquire inapparent infection from vast animal reservoirs of this organism? There have been numerous demonstrations of cross protection between closely related species and between widely disparate groups of organisms in the laboratory. Among the parasites there is overwhelming evidence of cross protection between the tick-borne piroplasms and malaria, between different species and genera of hookworms, between different species of tapeworms and schistosomes, in fact in almost all systems that have been studied, and the principle is being exploited to develop parasitic vaccines using heterologous infections of low pathogenicity in the same way as Jenner developed the smallpox vaccine[5].

The above examples involve the normal immunological responses of cross protection by stimulating either cell-mediated or antibody responses. The response can be either specific or much more generalized, for example in experimental systems BCG protects not only against tuberculosis but it gives good immunization against many different parasites. This type of non-specific immunization results from infection with a wide variety of organisms and efforts are being made to exploit this principle for protective immunization against parasitic disease[6]. There are even wider implications in these non-specific stimuli; with helminth infections there is almost invariably a marked increase in eosinophils in the circulation or in the tissues, and Fernex and Sternby[7] have argued that the increase in mast cells may be one of the reasons for the major differences in atherosclerosis and myocardial infarction in Africans compared with Europeans. When people of African origin lose their parasites and become 'civilized' they begin to acquire the same degenerative diseases that affect the more developed countries. Similar indirect effects of parasites may account for the differences in other conditions such as asthma. We are only beginning to understand some of these interrelationships. Perhaps we should take a more kindly view of the organisms in our environment and before we spend vast sums on trying to produce a sterile Utopia we might try and understand their evolutionary significance and their rôle as symbionts which might be conferring more benefit than harm, especially in rural communities where man is close to nature.

References

1. Nelson, G. S. (1970). The epidemiological significance of intraspecific variations in helminths of medical importance; with particular reference to *Trichinella* and *Schistosoma*. In: H. D. Srivastava Commemoration Volume, Singh, K. S. Y. Tandan, B. K. (Editors), pp. 19–25. (Izatnagar, India: Indian Veterinary and Research Institute)
2. Godfrey, D. G. (1978). Identification of economically important parasites. *Nature*, 273, 600
3. Medical Research Council Symposium (1977). Humidifier Fever. *Thorax*, 32, 653
4. Knight, R. and Worms, M. J. (1972). An outbreak of cercarial dermatitis in Britain. Demonstration. *Trans. R. Soc. Trop. Med. Hyg.*, 66, 21
5. Nelson, G. S. (1974). Zooprophylaxis with special reference to schistosomiasis and filariasis. *Parasitic Zoonoses: Clinical and Experimental Studies.* pp. 273–285. (New York: Academic Press Inc.)
6. Cox, F. E. G. (1978). Specific and non specific immunity against parasitic infections. *Nature*, 273, 623
7. Fernex, M. and Sternby, N. H. (1964). Mast cells and coronary heart disease. Relationship between numbers of mast cells in the myocardium, severity of coronary atherosclerosis and myocardial infarction in an autopsy series of 672 cases. *Acta path. Microbiol. Scand.* 62, 525

2
Insects (Hexapoda)

J. W. MAUNDER

INTRODUCTION

The insects are both an ancient[1] and a numerous[2] group of animals. Their long phase of adaptive radiation from their origins in the Palaeozoic, and their flexible lines of evolution have produced a modern insect fauna of extreme diversity. Yet nearly all insects retain clear evidence of their origins and relationships.

The insects retain, at least in the adult form, the protective chitinous exoskeleton and tubular jointed legs which proclaim their membership of the Phylum Arthropoda and their consequent kinship with crustaceans, spiders, centipedes, ticks and the like.

Amongst present-day animals the Class Insecta is probably most closely allied with the Myriapoda, a group containing the centipedes and millipedes[3]. Insects differ from these and from all other arthropods by having the adult body clearly divided into three sections, head, thorax and abdomen. Other groups may divide into two sections, for example spiders, mites and ticks which are divided only into a cephalothorax and an abdomen.

Adult insects have reduced the number of legs to six only, situated on the thorax. Other adult arthropods almost without exception have eight or more.

Most, but not all, adult insects possess compound eyes and one or two pairs of wings. Neither of these features appears in any other invertebrate group.

Origins of parasitism in insects

The habit of parasitism has developed on numerous independent occasions during the long history of insects. Some Orders have no parasitic members, these being usually the more primitive groups. Others have occasional examples of it, as in the Coleoptera (beetles) where, despite being by far the largest Order of insects, very few species are parasitic. Yet other Orders have a very substantial proportion of their species adopting the habit; the

11

Hymenoptera (wasps, ants and bees) being such an example. Of the 29 Orders recognized by Imms[4] four are exclusively parasitic, these being the Mallophaga (biting lice), the Anoplura (sucking lice), the Siphonaptera (the fleas) and the Strepsiptera (considered by some to be aberrant beetles). The hosts used by parasitic insects are extremely diverse. Frequently other insects are used as host. The general subject is treated by Askew[5].

Parasitism affecting man

Since man is a comparative newcomer, very few insects have as yet adapted to exploit him directly as a host species. A number of other species parasitize man more or less accidentally as a departure from their usual choice of host and in such cases the insects concerned may not be able to complete their normal development.

Parasites and microcarnivores

No sharp boundaries exist between parasites, commensals and carnivores. A mosquito biting man, even though feeding on man by preference, is regarded as a microcarnivore. A louse living on man and sucking his blood in an essentially similar manner is rightly regarded as a parasite.

However, intermediate conditions exist. A bed bug may bite man far less frequently than a mosquito and spend very little time on his person and yet be regarded as parasitic because it lives in our houses. Thus certain insects are regarded as parasites mainly because it is traditional to do so. Other insects may have various degrees of association with man less intimate than complete parasitism. Busvine's book[6] is a useful and practical guide to such insects.

Vector capacity in parasitic insects

Insects parasitic on man may not only cause disease directly, they may also carry and transfer other diseases. A person having lice has the disease *pediculosis*, but if the lice are carrying the bacterium *Rickettsia prowazeki* he will probably have typhus as well.

Since parasitic insects live in a sheltered environment provided by man's body or his home, they are less at the mercy of weather conditions and less concerned than free-living species with climatic considerations. In consequence, they tend to be geographically widespread, living wherever man can live, and tend to be just as effective vectors of disease in temperate climates as in tropical, and sometimes more so. The insect vectors most powerfully affecting Western man are the parasitic vectors. Typhus and European relapsing fever can be very efficiently carried by lice in colder countries as can plague by fleas, simply because man himself is providing warmth and shelter to his parasitic vectors of disease.

The subject of disease transmission by insect vectors in general is covered by Herms' book[7], though, like all textbooks of general medical entomology, it has a very considerable tropical bias.

THE ANOPLURA (SUCKING LICE)

All three types of human louse are members of this Order, which is an homogeneous group of 500 known species, all haematophagous ectoparasites of mammals. All spend the whole of their life-cycle on the host, never voluntarily leaving it except for another animal of the same species in contact. All are strongly host-specific, for not only is each species usually associated with one host animal alone, but often will occur on one part only of that one host. Spread is invariably by contact, either social or sexual.

Zoologically there is little remarkable about human lice. They have better developed eyes than most animal lice but otherwise they strongly conform to the norms of their order. They too have no food but blood and have their entire life cycle on the host, never voluntarily leaving except for another human being. Human lice too have preferences for certain parts of the body, and are spread by contact, social or sexual.

Nor is there anything remarkable about the physical effects of lice. In man and animals the effects include direct toxic effects of injected saliva, allergic sensitization to saliva and faeces, and the possibility of the insects acting as vectors of yet more serious disease. Each louse on a human being, and there may be several hundred, feeds five or six times daily and injects saliva into the bloodstream on each occasion. All of us who have carried experimental infestations can testify that the direct effects include a general weariness combined with dull aching of legs and feet. An irritable and pessimistic mood develops and the temperature may rise slightly. The lousy feel lousy.

Prolonged biting results in sensitization, occasionally in as short a time as two weeks but often delayed for several months. With sensitization, irritation from the bites, previously minimal, becomes severe, occasioning loss of sleep and leading to scratching and sometimes secondary infection. In sensitized individuals the louse faeces (a copious black powder) may cause symptoms reminiscent of hay fever when breathed in, and intense irritation if they fall into the eyes.

Much more remarkable than the biology or physical effects of lice are the psychological effects engendered in both sufferer and beholder. Lice can cause emotive and often illogical reactions in both groups. The mere possession of lice may cause a substantial drop in social status and may easily cause the sufferer, especially if young, to regard himself as an innately inferior person. This has its counterpart in those who have contact with the lousy, for society seems to have a need to humiliate those with lice. In effect the lousy are often punished for lowering the social tone of the neighbourhood, school or family.

In Western countries the disease vector effect of human lice is minimal under normal circumstances, being confined to spreading bacterial secondary infection. If normal standards of life were lowered by military or natural disasters louse-born disease could soon return. Our freedom from relapsing fever, classical typhus and other serious diseases must in part depend on our continuing to keep lice under control.

The relationships and higher classification of the Order are treated by Ke Chung Kim and Ludwig[8], the host relationships are reviewed by Hopkins[9] and the biology of human lice by Buxton[10].

Crab or pubic lice

The louse *Phthirus pubis** is such a typical member of its Order that it causes little surprise to the entomologist, although frequently affording most unpleasant surprises to those with whom it chooses to dwell. Its distribution on the body is determined by characteristics of body hair, its preference being for widely-spaced coarse hair. Thus, apart from its favourite site amongst the pubic hair, it may also be found on hairy legs, in axillary hair and, more rarely, in beards. In infants the lice occur occasionally in eyelashes and around the edges of head hair.

The louse (Figure 2.1) is an unenergetic insect spending much of its time at the base of a single hair. Repeated biting on the same spot may produce the

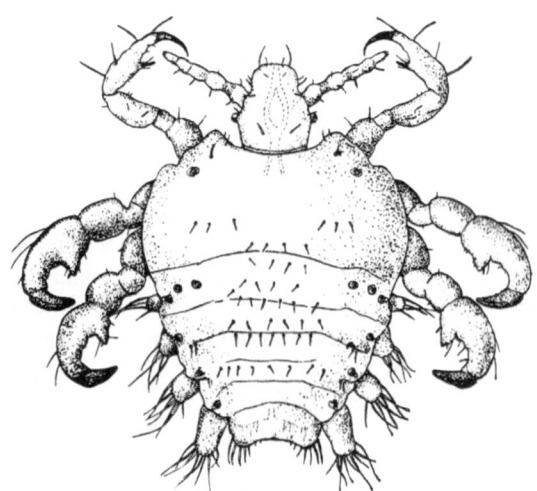

Figure 2.1 *Phthirus pubis*, crab louse, female, ×64. (From Patton, W. S. and Cragg, F. W. *A Textbook of Medical Entomology*, 1913)

* The accepted first description of the genus was printed as *Pthirus* due, it is said, to a printer's error. Some purists use this spelling contrary to classical derivation and common usage.

blue spots (*maculae cerulae*) so often mentioned in textbooks but these are really much rarer than the books seem to imply. So well camouflaged is this louse that it is easy to stare straight at it without seeing it, for they can assume a colour which blends with that of the skin. Eggs, which hatch in eight days, are glued to the hair. The young louse is mature in seven days and lives a further three weeks, the females laying about five eggs a day.

Spread is by contact, usually but not necessarily sexual. When the sufferer discovers the creatures the infestation is usually already some weeks old. Although the public lavatory seat used the previous week will be blamed, the real cause will usually be the sexual contact two or three months before.

As with most things of which people are ashamed, they are much commoner than usually realized. Unfortunately the doctor, a respected figure, is frequently one of the last people the patient would willingly tell and self-treatment is the rule. Fortunately modern veterinary flea powders are usually effective and harmless, but fly sprays, paraffin, petrol and old wives' remedies are not. The most effective treatment is with lotions containing 0.5% malathion or carbaryl. All of these lotions kill both eggs and lice in a few seconds so that a single application is all that is needed, though a second treatment one week after the first is usually recommended. The lotions may be washed off after half-an-hour, but are safe enough to leave on indefinitely.

Of the older preparations those containing gamma-benzene hexachloride have high patient acceptability. This is a slow insecticide which should not be washed off for six hours. As it is not ovicidal applications should be repeated weekly for three weeks. Gamma-benzene hexachloride is not thought to be as safe as more modern insecticides.

Powders are not as effective as lotions as less intimate contact with the insects is achieved. Those who prefer powders may find 2% gamma-benzene hexachloride acceptable, but not ovicidal. Four applications over nine days are needed to be sure that newly-hatched nymphs are killed. Shampoos have no place in pubic louse control.

Failure in control is usually due to inadequate application; all hairy areas below the neck should be treated. Shaving the pubic areas is unnecessary.

The rare cases of lice on eyelashes may be dealt with by gently removing accessible lice with forceps and carefully touching each egg with a fine brush dipped in one of the ovicidal lotions.

The body louse

The condition is caused by the louse *Pediculus humanus humanus* (Figure 2.2) which has abandoned the ancestral habits of the group by laying eggs on clothing next to the skin. Seams on the inner side of underclothes are considered particularly desirable. The louse only visits the skin to obtain its blood meals. Eggs are laid very close to the skin and hatch in seven days if kept continuously at skin temperature. If the temperature is lower for part or all of the

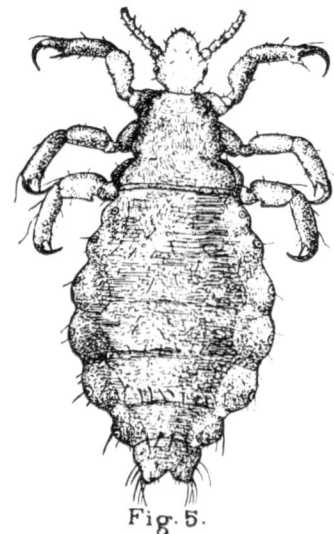

Fig. 5.

Figure 2.2   *Pediculus humanus humanus*, body louse, female, ×20. (From Patton, W. S. and Cragg, F. W. *A Textbook of Medical Entomology*, 1913)

time, hatching takes longer, but all eggs must hatch or die within 20 days. The young louse must feed on blood within about 36 hours, but this usually presents it with no problems. Empty eggshells remain attached to the cloth and are not usually removed by subsequent washing. Such eggs, or dead ones, can confuse a diagnosis based on the presence of eggs alone.

Under favourable circumstances the young louse becomes mature in seven days, moulting three times on the way. The extremely delicate cast skins produced may fly about, and were perhaps the origin of the erroneous idea that lice can be blown from person to person. In fact viable lice never let go of the clothing except for another human being or his clothing in contact, or unless the host dies or runs a quite exceptional temperature.

Female lice can lay six to eight eggs each day for 30 days, but few lice live this long as injury due to scratching usually intervenes. Injured lice do not recover.

Of all the 500 species of Anoplura this is the only one which can be discarded by the host at will. If the clothing is removed so are the lice, and continued existence for them depends on the same clothing being worn continuously, or at least for the greater part of each day.

Patients with body lice usually conceal the condition when visiting their doctors by changing their clothing. The condition may be suspected by the presence of heavily bitten areas which may approximately follow the outlines of an undervest or the seams of other clothing. Typically each bite raises a very small red papule which may weep a little. Bitten areas become swollen and eventually permanently hardened and darkened if biting continues for years. The latter condition is known as Vagabonds' disease, more tactfully described as *morbus errorum*.

When actual lice are discovered on the clothing of people brought to casualty departments or discovered as a result of home visiting, a disproportionate degree of consternation often results. In bright light the lice will not transfer to anyone handling lousy clothing and the only precaution needed is to prevent one's own clothing from touching it. Injured or aged lice might drop from clothing, but such lice, being too weak to maintain a hold, are dying and more alarming than dangerous.

Distinction needs to be made between dirtiness and lousiness in many practical situations. Clothing may be deloused by being put dry into a tumble drier for five minutes as suggested by Maunder[11], following which it may safely be sent to a conventional laundry or even be returned dirty but louse-free to the patient. Alternatively clothing may be fumigated with methyl bromide for 12 hours or washed in water hotter than 60 °C. The patient may be treated with lotions such as 0.5% malathion or with dusts (e.g. 5% carbaryl in talc, 40 g per clothed adult), though it is unusual for viable lice to remain on people after removal of the clothing. Restoration of normal laundering of clothes ends a body louse infestation.

Head lice

The human head louse *Pediculus humanus capitis* has been the cause of sufficient concern in recent years throughout the Western world to justify the inclusion of a separate chapter on its biology and control.

Animal lice

Animal lice cannot establish an infestation on man. Nevertheless animal lice do sometimes transfer onto human beings handling animals. They are generally of no significance to man, although several are important veterinary pests of animals and birds.

HETEROPTERA (TRUE BUGS)

The classification of the true bugs remains the subject of controversy, and some still place the entire group with the related Homoptera (the plant lice) as a single Order, the Hemiptera.

The Heteroptera all have piercing and sucking mouthparts but the range of food utilized is wide. Many are phytophagous, others predatory. Bloodsucking forms often attack other insects but a few have become microcarnivores preying on birds or mammals, and of these some have crossed the boundary from predation to parasitism. Many of the group can inflict painful defence bites on man, even if not of a bloodsucking species. A general account of the order is given by Poisson[12].

Of over 50 Families recognized, only two contain members regarded as parasites of man.

The Cimicidae (bed bugs)

The bed bugs form an exclusively parasitic group whose sole food is the blood of warm-blooded animals. Their parasitic adaptations are comparatively slight, the loss of wings being the most obvious, and few species make any attempt to cling to the host. Three species have man as a primary host but only one of these is found in temperate countries.

Cimex lectularius (The common bed bug)

The common or temperate bed bug, *Cimex lectularius* (Figure 2.3) is cosmopolitan in distribution although more frequent in cooler countries. The

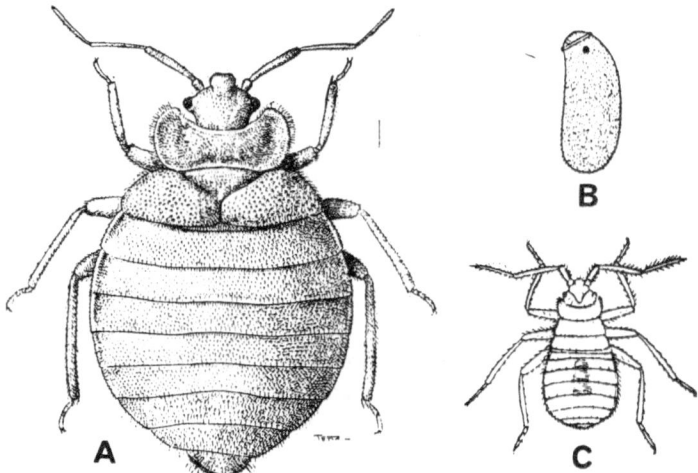

Figure 2.3 *Cimex lectularius*, the common bed bug: A, dorsal view of male adult; B, egg; C, newly hatched nymph (not all to same scale). (From K. G. V. Smith (ed.) *Insects and other Arthropods of Medical Importance,* 1973. With permission from the editor and the Trustees of the British Museum (Natural History))

normal host is man but rare infestations of chickens, bats and laboratory rodents have been recorded.

Feeding takes place in the hour or two just before dawn when the bugs leave their homes in crevices of walls and furniture, to seek their sleeping victims. Biting is most frequent on the head, hands and arms of the victim but can occur anywhere. During feeding the previously greatly flattened insect swells up with blood but immediately diuretic hormones act to reduce the excess liquid taken aboard. Liquid urine (unusual in insects) is eliminated via the rectum leaving small brown or black marks on sheets etc. It is these marks which give the creature its name, for it is extremely rare to find a bug in a bed, although they may be found in the bedstead itself and sometimes under buttons on mattresses. The earlier name 'wall louse' was in some ways more appropriate, for their homes are often under loose wallpaper or in cracks in walls or woodwork. Defaecation marks are often found on walls and the cast skins of the creatures at the foot of infested walls.

Eggs are oval with a cap at one end. They are pearly in colour, about 1 mm in length and glued to rough surfaces in or near the crevices in which the adults live. The new hatched young are miniatures of the adult and moult five times before becoming mature, when they will be about 5 mm in length. The bug is oval in outline, flattened from top to bottom, with six prominent legs but no wings and dark brown in colour.

Each bug feeds about every third night in warm weather, less frequently as the night temperature falls, and ceases to feed if the room temperature falls below 10 °C. Their nuisance value is therefore highly seasonal except where central heating keeps them active all winter. Well-fed bugs can starve for over 150 days. The life cycle takes from four to seven months and individual bugs can live more than a year.

Biting reaction is very variable. A few people show no reaction but extremely severe responses may occur in others. Relief for one or two nights may be obtained by sleeping with the light on. Repellents are very unsatisfactory.

Bed bugs spread in furniture and belongings moved from house to house. The presence of the bugs can often be detected by spraying a pyrethroid flyspray into suspicious cracks. This will not kill them but may irritate them enough to make them leave their homes in the day-time.

In few places in the Western world are bugs now a major problem but neither are they rare, and in some places they are making a comeback, which is presumed to be due to the increased use of prefabricated materials for housing. This provides the crevices so beloved by this insect.

Although bed bugs carry no diseases their effects in the realm of social medicine may be considerable. Being so strongly linked with structurally second-rate buildings and with low standards of hygiene, infected property tends to be occupied by the most uncaring, inadequate or helpless members of the community. As Busvine[6] points out, bed bugs may not only be typical of slums but actually a cause of them.

Being both naturally tolerant of insecticides and deeply hidden in narrow crevices, bugs are difficult to control. Persistent insecticides applied as sprays by experts hold the best promise of success followed by thorough structural repair and redecoration.

The ecology of the bed bug is described by Johnson[13]. The important monograph on the entire Family Cimicidae by Usinger[14] should be consulted by those requiring further information.

The tropical bed bugs

Two other bed bugs have man as the prime host. *Cimex hemipterus* is found throughout the tropics and *Leptocimex bousti* is confined to tropical West Africa. Neither species can establish itself outside the tropics, although *C. hemipterus* is found in Florida.

Animal bed bugs

In Europe the pigeon bug *Cimex columbarius* has been known to invade houses from nesting sites in roof spaces and *Oeciacus hirundinis*, the martin bug, does likewise. Both can be found on the outside of houses, which the true bed bug never frequents. In North America, *O. hirundinis* is replaced by *O. vicarius*. Bat bugs have also been known to infest houses. As all members of the family strongly resemble each other an expert identification is desirable if a bed bug infestation has markedly unusual features or does not respond to expert control measures.

The Reduviidae (The assassin bugs)

Most members of this large family are insectivorous (hence their name) but the Subfamily Triatominae are suckers of vertebrate blood and are of great importance in tropical medicine. Some temperate region triatomines are capable of infesting houses in a very similar manner to bed bugs and so qualify as facultative and opportunistic parasites of man. All are comparatively large insects, with winged adults and a comparatively long life cycle. No sharp distinction can be made between them and the non-parasitic members, for the two states merge into one another.

Examples include the China bed bug, *Triatoma protracta,* common on the Pacific sea coast of the United States, and the Mexican bed bug *Triatoma sanguisuma* in the south of the country. Usinger[15] has published a comprehensive account of the North American species.

An interesting member of the family is the masked bed bug hunter, *Reduvius personatus.* This bug is also found in Britain and Europe as well as in North America. Normally it hunts and kills the common human bed bug and is thus found in houses. If disturbed it can inflict a defence bite said to be one of the most painful of all insect bites.

The defence bites of reduviids contain toxins which increase the pain whereas feeding bites are initially painless. The bites of some species can cause complications, including cutaneous growths resembling papillomas, which may persist for many months.

SIPHONAPTERA (FLEAS)

The fleas constitute a well-defined and distinct order of insects comprising some 2700 species. Their interaction with man can be complex, for their life cycles are always complicated by non-parasitic larval stages and nearly always by the necessary presence of a warm-blooded host other than man. Indeed, it is probable that man is not the preferred host for any species of flea. Even the so-called 'human' flea may be regarded as being more properly a parasite of earth-burrowing carnivorous mammals such as foxes, its presence in association with man being opportunistic.

Fleas are essentially insects associated with the nests and burrows, for it is here that the eggs hatch, the omnivorous larvae scavenge for food and the pupae, wrapped in silken cocoons, undergo the momentous metamorphosis which results in the adult flea (Figure 2.4). Often, too, it is in the nest or burrow that the majority of adult fleas are found, for in many species the bloodsucking adults are but hit-and-run raiders of the resting host, feeding quickly and jumping off again. So it is that nomadic animals, such as cattle or apes, do not have flea parasites unless man forces them to be of fixed abode by shutting them in stables or zoos, when they may acquire flea species not natural to them.

In nature a single flea species may be so host-specific that it is confined to one host alone, or may be so catholic as to be able to breed in association with numerous and diverse host species. Much of the specificity is determined by the conditions provided by the hosts' dwelling place—individual fleas may often get onto and even bite the 'wrong' hosts, but breeding requires a suitable place as well as a suitable host.

Recognition of fleas

The adult is generally encountered and not easily captured undamaged. For a loose flea, dabbing with a wet bar of soap is sometimes recommended, but often even such simple apparatus is not to hand and the creature suffers instant death under a thumb or rolled-up newspaper. When recovering fleas from the fur of animals with a fine tooth comb the escape of the insects can be inhibited by slightly dampening the fur first. However mangled the corpse of a flea may be, a professional entomologist can usually identify it, so damaged specimens are well worth submitting for examination. It is helpful if several specimens can be sent as some identification procedures involve the partial destruction of the specimen or are facilitated by both sexes being present. Specimens are preferably sent preserved in 70% alcohol, but may also be sent dry[16]. Those wishing to attempt their own identifications will find Busvine[6] useful in the beginning and Smith[17] when more expert, but the matter is fraught with difficulty. In practice, however, identification of the host animal involved is usually an easy matter and gives reasonably reliable evidence of the flea probably present.

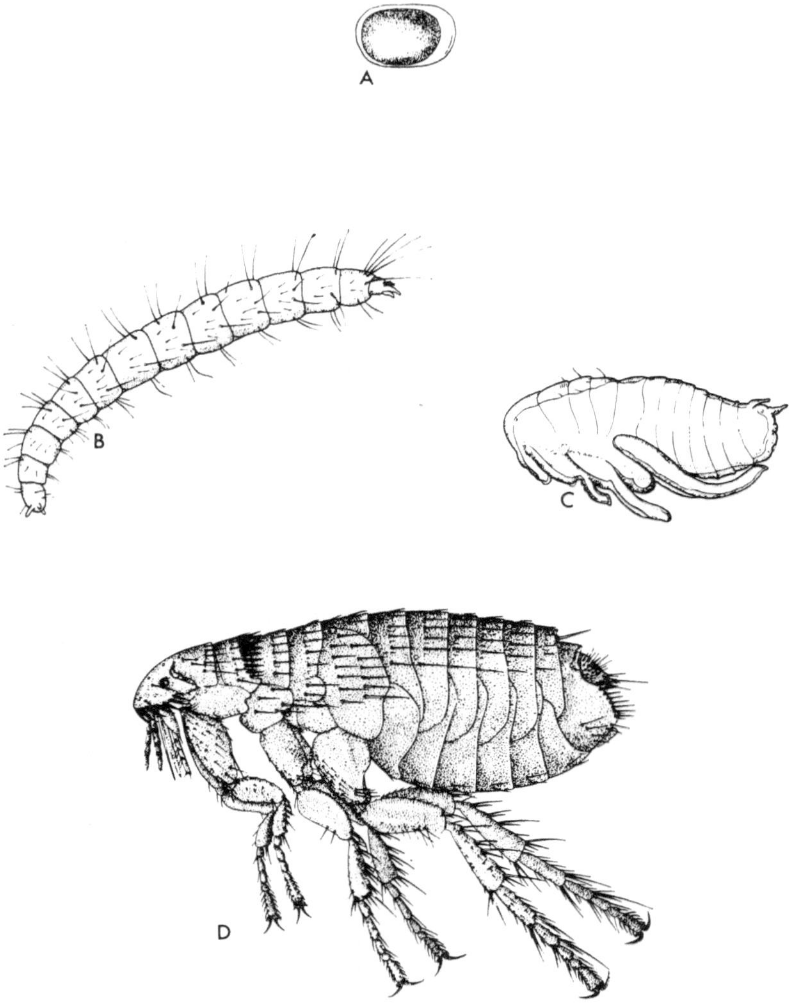

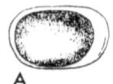

Figure 2.4 *Xenopsylla cheopis*, the plague flea: A, egg; B, larva; C, pupa; D, *Ctenocephalides felis felis*, the cat flea, female. (From K. G. V. Smith (ed.) *Insects and other Arthropods of Medical Importance*, 1973. With permission from the editor and the Trustees of the British Museum (Natural History))

Cosmopolitan domestic species

Due to the activities of man a number of species of flea may now be found in human dwellings in any region of the world.

Pulex irritans (The human flea)

This flea, *Pulex irritans*, is the only temperate flea able to live and breed in association with man as the sole host. It is usually a bedroom dweller, having a preference for cool, damp and dirty conditions. Larvae and fleas may live in human beds, being commonest where unwashed blankets are used without sheets. It can also breed in cracks of dirty floors and can use other primary hosts including dogs and cats. The flea may travel some distance on a person before biting, so bite marks may occur anywhere on the body. If the bite occurs under clothing, specks of blood may stain the clothes at that point as the flea when feeding to repletion discharges almost unchanged blood from its anus.

Drier, warmer and cleaner homes have made this flea virtually extinct in Western countries save in some areas of bad housing and hygiene, usually rural.

In Western and Southern parts of North America a very closely related flea of similar habits co-exists with *P. irritans*. This flea is also known as the 'human' flea, but is scientifically named *P. simulans*.

Ctenocephalides felis (The cat flea)

Ctenocephalides felis is the outstanding nuisance flea of the modern Western World. Many factors have combined to favour it in recent years including better central heating, undisturbed fitted carpets and the greater licence granted to pet animals. It is also the commonest flea found in association with dogs.

This flea spends more time on the host than does the human flea, yet still the great majority of adult fleas are off the host, lying quietly in some place to which the host regularly returns. These fleas will bite man readily when deprived of access to the usual hosts, but do not like to travel under clothing. Bites, therefore, tend to be at relatively exposed sites, the lower leg and hands and wrists being particularly favoured. Children who are allowed pets in bed with them may be bitten on the trunk, occasionally causing alarm when parents conclude that the bites are manifestations of infectious disease.

The flea is very common. Few cats will escape having it at some time, and it is not uncommon in dogs. It is the usual invertebrate host, and vector of, the dog tapeworm *Dipyllidium caninum*. This worm also affects cats and children; not serious but not welcome (see Chapter 8).

Ctenocephalides canis (The dog flea)

Ctenocephalides canis is closely related to the cat flea. The two species are easily confused, usually leading to false positive identifications of dog fleas, which are altogether rarer than cat fleas, especially in warmer climates. The life style, habits and effects on man are closely similar in the two species, although the dog flea needs to be the more hungry before biting man. Dog fleas can also live on cats.

Xenopsylla cheopis (The plague flea)

The preferred host for *Xenopsylla cheopis* is the ship rat, *Rattus rattus*, also known as the black rat or roof rat. The flea is also known as the tropical rat flea, but is by no means confined to the tropics. (Indeed, the plague itself has tended to be subtropical and warm-temperate rather than strictly tropical.) The flea can also breed in association with other rodents, including the brown rat, *Rattus norvegicus*. If deprived of rodent blood, for example when the rats are dying of disease, it will readily bite man. *Rattus rattus* (and its flea) was formerly much more common in domestic situations as it likes thatched roofs and bare rafters, being very much a climbing animal.

Other rodent fleas

The brown rat, also known as the Norwegian rat, is the commonest domestic rat nearly everywhere in the Western world. Its usual flea, *Nosopsyllus fasciatus*, is often found in houses especially after rodent control operations unaccompanied by insecticide treatments. Only under extreme starvation will an occasional one bite man—most would rather die first.

The flea of the house mouse is *Leptopsylla segnis*, which is unusual in being quite blind. It spends nearly all its adult life actually on the host, but may also be found free in houses, especially if the mice are being killed. It rarely bites man.

Bird fleas

A number of fleas normally associated with birds will bite man when unable to find their usual host.

Ceratophyllus gallinae is commonly found on birds likely to nest in or near human dwellings. It is called the hen flea, but although found on domestic fowl it is more frequent on wild birds including pigeons, martins and other peridomestic species. In Britain it is the next most serious biting nuisance after the cat flea[18]. It often invades downwards from old nests in roof spaces, and is in consequence primarily a bedroom biter.

Ceratophyllus columbae has similar habits but is usually found only on pigeons.

Endoparasitic fleas

A number of fleas have developed the habit of being permanently attached to the skin of the host throughout their adult life. The poultry flea *Echidnophaga gallinacea* and the rabbit flea *Spilopsyllus cuniculi* are examples of considerable veterinary importance and both may attach to humans coming into close contact with the hosts, causing some annoyance.

The habit is further developed with the jigger flea (also known as the chigoe) which becomes effectively endoparasitic, with more serious consequences to affected human beings. This flea, *Tunga penetrans*, is strictly tropical. It is found in both Old and New Worlds, although rare as yet in Asia. Visitors to areas where it is found can easily acquire them, especially if they walk barefoot along paths used by farm and domestic animals.

The adult female flea attaches to the skin which soon becomes swollen and ulcerated. She becomes buried in the skin and swells to many times her original size. Only the tip of her abdomen protrudes from the skin and from this fall many hundreds of eggs. Secondary infection is always present, sometimes of such severity that amputation has to be resorted to. The feet are most commonly affected, but any part of the body may be chosen.

The fleas are easily removed at an early stage with a sterile needle, but by the time visitors to the tropics return home and subsequently seek medical advice the fleas are usually approaching full size, about 5 mm in diameter. As the developed female consists virtually entirely of hugely enlarged ovaries in a membranous abdomen the insect can rarely be removed whole and in any case no longer resembles a conventional flea. Identification is usually by means of the masses of oval eggs visible by microscopic examination. The cavities left by flea removal need very careful cleaning if flea debris is not to remain and delay healing.

Principles of control of domestic fleas

With the exception of the human flea, human beings are somewhat distasteful to fleas and are usually only bitten as an emergency measure. They become most troublesome when the death or removal of the normal host leaves a flea colony deprived of its usual nourishment. Flea control measures are a frequent adjunct to vertebrate pest control programmes.

Fleas are essentially an infestation of a place occupied by a host as distinct from an infestation of the host. For example, a typical cat flea colony may consist of some 5000 individuals, distributed (at any one time) as follows:

—adult fleas on the cat	25
—adult fleas off the cat	500
—pupae in cocoons	500
—larvae in floors and bedding	3000
—eggs	1000

Clearly, control measures solely directed against insects on the cat are unlikely to be successful, so treatment of the whole environment is necessary. Fleas in cocoons are protected against insecticides so that either reasonably persistent compounds should be used, or the whole treatment repeated every week or two for six months. Repellents are of little use against permanent contact with fleas as although they may keep them at bay for a day or two, eventually the insects become hungry enough to overcome them. However, the medical practitioner making house calls to homes suspected of harbouring fleas may find a little dimethyl phthalate smeared on his socks keeps the invaders away.

DIPTERA (FLIES)

The very large order of two-winged flies contains many species of medical importance including virtually all of the flying haematophagous insects. The parasitic habit was absent from ancestral forms but has developed many times as the order has diversified, being found in widely variable presentations amongst the more advanced groups. Although there are many flies parasitic in the adult form, none attacks man, so that we have to deal only with parasitic larvae (Figure 2.5).

The infestation of living vertebrates with living fly larvae is termed myiasis. The condition is so variable in terms of the parasites involved, in variations of

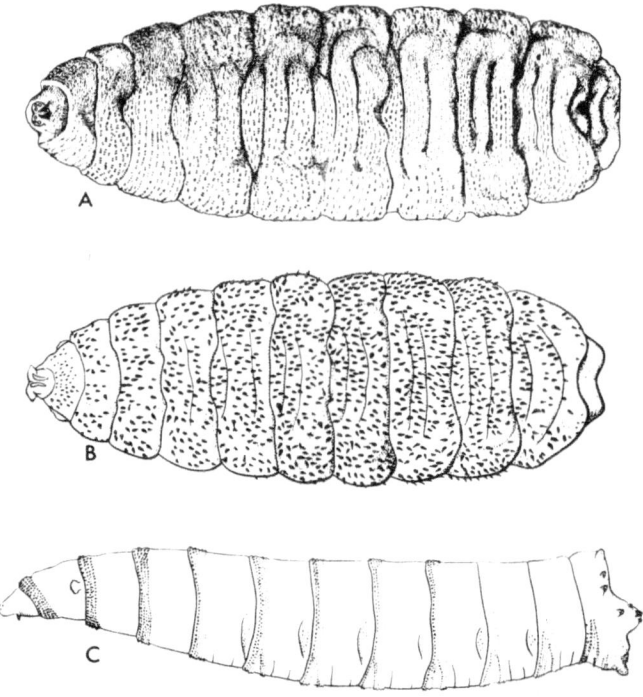

Figure 2.5 Third instar larvae of Calliphoridae: A, *Cordylobia anthropophaga* (Tumbu-fly), ventral; B, *Cordylobia (Strasisia) rodhaini,* ventral; C, *Cochliomyia (Callitroga) macellaria,* lateral. (From K. G. V. Smith (ed.) *Insects and other Arthropods of Medical Importance,* 1973. With permission from the editor and the Trustees of the British Museum (Natural History))

life cycles, and in mode and site of attack that it is difficult to give a logical and coherent account of the phenomenon. Zumpt[19] has a very significant monograph on the subject but has confined his examples to the Old World. Scott[20] deals with the New World and Lee[21] with Australia.

The primary classification adopted here is into furuncular, traumatic and body cavity myiases. This has admitted shortcomings but may have advantages for Western clinicians who are unlikely to see myiasis frequently.

Recognition of dipterous larvae

Maggots recovered from human beings are unlikely to be mistaken for other than dipterous larvae, but the recognition of the exact species involved can be a matter of extreme difficulty even for a professional entomologist. Those wishing to attempt their own identifications may find the key of Oldroyd and Smith[22] very useful.

When submitting larvae for identification the task of the entomologist can be made much easier by the observance of a few simple points. If larvae of more than one size are present then send some of each size. If numerous larvae are present some live ones are worth submitting, but if only one or a few are available they should be preserved in 70% alcohol. In the absence of an exact 70% alcohol, neat gin or vodka are reasonable alternatives, although causing some swelling of specimens. Under no circumstances should formalin or any preservative containing formaldehyde ever be used for preserving larvae. It is very helpful if a list of countries or states visited by the patient during the previous year can be supplied and also reasonably full clinical details concerning the recovery of the maggot.

Furuncular myiasis

The term describes a condition where a boil-like lesion is present, normally containing only one larva (which may be of considerable size). According to species the larva may have developed *in situ* or may have spent many months migrating through the body before forming the furuncle as a site of exit.

Warble fly myiasis

The larvae of the warble flies are grubs as opposed to maggots (i.e. the body has its greatest diameter midway along its length instead of at its posterior end). The grubs normally develop in cattle, having hatched from eggs laid on hairs and penetrating the skin. After nearly a year of complex migration within the host the grubs move to the skin of the back to form a large swelling or warble, out of which the mature larva eventually bursts its way. Pupation then takes place on the ground.

In man the life cycle is essentially similar. The wanderings of the grub may include the intestines and nervous system, causing at best discomfort and often excruciating pain. Curiously, serious after-effects are rare at this stage, but when the grub is mature it has difficulty in escaping from human beings and may then cause very grave damage. In cattle an upward migration brings it to the back, but in man may bring it into the head. A warble forming on the shoulders or head external to the skull is unpleasant enough, but a larva trapped in the skull cavities can cause death.

Three species are particularly important. *Hypoderma lineatum*, the lesser cattle warble, is found in the United States, parts of Canada and also in Europe and Asia. The larger cattle warble *H. bovis* has a range extending to the northern limits of cattle farming. *H. diana* is found only in Europe where its normal host is deer. A number of other warbles are found on rare occasions in man (see also Chapter 9).

Bot fly myiasis

The parasitic part of the life cycle of bot flies differs from warble flies in that after entry through the host's skin all development proceeds in the subdermal tissues without migration. A boil-like lesion forms at the site of entry and as in warbles the mature larva breaks out from this, falls to the ground and pupates without further feeding. Human infestations with bots originating in temperate regions are very unusual. When they do occur they usually involve flies of the genus *Cuterebra* whose normal hosts include rodents and rabbits. The grubs are large and often formidably spiny. Nevertheless they do not penetrate deeply and are easily removed.

Much more frequent in many Western surgeries are tropical bot flies infesting those who have travelled recently in tropical regions. Two species are of major importance.

Dermatobia hominis is the New World human bot fly. It is an important cattle pest of the tropical Americas including Mexico. The female fly has the curious habit of laying eggs by proxy! She captures a female cattle-biting mosquito, attaches her eggs to it and then releases it. The next time the mosquito feeds the warmth of the host hatches the fly eggs which then penetrate unbroken skin to initiate the myiasis. If man is the target of the mosquito he becomes infected, although cattle are the principal hosts. In human beings the larvae take about 50 days to become mature. The lesions can be very painful but are rarely serious.

The Old World human bot fly is *Cordylobia anthropophaga*, restricted to tropical and southern Africa. It too avoids laying directly on human beings. The usual oviposition site is sandy soil near human habitations, especially if contaminated with urine. It is not infrequent for eggs to be laid in clothing hung out to dry after being washed carelessly. After hatching the larvae can wander for two weeks seeking a host. In man skin penetration is rapid and painless, but the resulting furuncle is very painful. The surrounding skin becomes hardened and the boil weeps a serous fluid. Systemic effects are not uncommon, with fever and malaise. Removal must be thorough, for any insect debris remaining in the cavity delays healing and ecourages secondary infection, which is a frequent complication with this species.

Traumatic myiasis

This term may be used to describe irregular lesions containing several, usually many, larvae. In the evolutionary sense this type of myiasis developed amongst flies whose larvae bred in carrion. Some developed the ability to utilize necrotic tissue and exudates from wounds in still living animals, and as a natural progression a number of species began to utilize both dead and living flesh as normal breeding material. A few species have become obligatory parasites unable to use any food but living flesh. None is a parasite of man exclusively.

An example of obligatory parasitism is provided by the celebrated New World screw worm, *Cochliomyia hominivorax*. The female seeks wounds, preferably suppurating ones. No wound is too small, even insect bites may be used. According to the size of the site a group of eggs is deposited varying from 10 to over 300. Hatching is rapid and the mass of larvae eat their way to full size in only four days, causing extensive open lesions. They then drop out to pupate. Unfortunately the fly sometimes regards an infected nasal cavity as a particularly fine wound. The resulting nasopharyngeal myiasis can only be described as appalling, often resulting in death.

The Old World screw worm, *Chrysomya bezziana*, is confined to tropical regions and is virtually never seen in Western countries.

The best-known obligatory parasite of the screw worm type in Europe is *Wohlfahrtia magnifica*, a fly also found in all other Palaeoarctic regions. Live young are produced, being dropped as a wriggling mass into wounds and also on occasion into nasal openings and ears. The umbilicus of newborn babies is a favoured site if available, and deaths have been recorded.

Facultative traumatic myiasis may be no less serious. Many species can be involved, usually in the genera *Lucillia* ('green blowflies'), *Calliphora* ('blue blowflies') and *Sarcophaga* (flesh flies). The wounds chosen are usually less fresh than with screw worms; ulcerated and necrotic tissues allow the maggots a good start before they move on to living flesh.

An old wound, perhaps already containing parasitic dipterous larvae, often attracts flies whose larvae are not strictly parasites but rather saprophytes. If enough dead material is present almost any carrion-breeding fly may be attracted. The presence of these non-parasitic larvae is sometimes called benign myiasis, for often they will eat out all trace of necrotic tissue leaving the wound free to heal. The effect has been deliberately utilized in times past. At least a dozen genera may be involved including houseflies (*Musca, Muscina* and *Fannia*), blowflies (*Lucillia, Phaenicia, Calliphora* and *Phormia*) and flesh flies (*Sarcophaga*).

Myiasis of gut and body cavities

The heterogeneous groups of conditions described in this section have in common their increasing rarity in Western countries. However, any breakdown in modern living conditions, as might be caused by natural disasters or by war, would rapidly augment their numbers.

Intestinal myiasis

True myiasis of the human gut is restricted to rare examples of dung-breeding flies laying eggs or live larvae around the anus, followed by penetration and existence (usually brief) in the rectum.

Several flies, especially within the Family Calliphoridae, will readily lay live larvae in very fresh human excrement, sometimes while it is in the very act of deposition. This has led to numerous false reports of intestinal myiasis.

Intestinal pseudomyiasis

If maggotty food is eaten, the larvae pass into and through the human gut. This is in no sense a true parasitism in that the larvae do not develop in any way and are often killed. Any surviving the entire passage through the intestines can usually only do so if severe disturbance of the digestion is already present.

Nevertheless, the presence of dipterous larvae in the gut will often cause great pain, accompanied by diarrhoea and vomiting. Sometimes the symptoms have been mistaken for those of appendicitis. Some larvae cause mechanical damage due to their spines and sharp mouth hooks. Mental symptoms resembling depression occur in a high proportion of cases, presumably due to some toxic effect of the larvae.

Continuous passing of maggots for months on end, as has been described in the literature, can only be due to continuous intake of contaminated food or to deliberate swallowing of maggots by the patient, as there is no way in which the maggots can multiply in human intestines.

The passage of fly larvae through the alimentary canal has been termed intestinal pseudomyiasis by Zumpt[19]. West[23] provides an introduction to the subject although his conclusions have not met with total acceptance.

Larvae may be ingested in flyblown meat, when any of the carrion-breeding flies may be involved. Other maggots may be present on dried or preserved foods including bacon, cheese and smoked fish. The cheese-skipper *Piophila casei* may be found on most such foods and is a common cause of trouble.

Contaminated water may yield the rat-tailed larvae of *Eristalis tenax* and over-ripe fruit larvae of *Drosophila* and *Hermetia*. Even root crops may harbour maggots, the carrot root fly *Psila rosae* being one example.

Cutaneous larva migrans

Flies of the genus *Gasterophilus*, normally obligatory enteric parasites of horses, occasionally affect man. Larvae penetrate the skin of the head or mouth of the horse, migrate to the stomach and re-emerge into the gut where they attach in a manner reminiscent of tapeworms.

In man the larva may penetrate the skin anywhere, but the larva can only wander through the skin leaving a bright red line of inflammation behind it. The larva never develops further and never penetrates to the gut as it does in the natural host.

Urinogenital myiasis

This may be of the traumatic type already referred to, or may be due to larvae living in the cavities without general invasion of the flesh. The lesser housefly *Fannia canicularis* and the latrine fly *Fannia scalaris* are the usual species encountered.

Eggs are presumably laid near the urinary orifice, newly hatched larvae then entering and finding the bladder, where they may cause damage to the wall and great discomfort. Passing maggots in the urine is particularly painful. Larvae can develop slowly in the bladder but rarely do so in the vagina. Mature larvae can be found there, but the possibility must be considered that they might have been put there. The introduction of insects, spiders, centipedes and the like into the vagina, presumably to gain extra attention, occurs sufficiently frequently for most medical entomologists to be able to give examples from their own professional experience.

Myiasis of the orbit

A number of flies have maggots which are obligatory parasites of the nasal cavities and sinuses of mammals. Two of these attack man with some frequency, but it is curious that both flies, of different genera, deposit larvae in the eyes rather than the nostrils of man. The female insects boldly fly up to the eye, striking the eyeball sharply with the abdomen and depositing a live-born larva. The larva never develops, but dies or is expelled in a day or two, and little harm is ever done. Vary rarely the maggots are laid in the nose, but even in this more natural site they do not develop and as a rule nothing worse than sinus irritation follows.

The two species usually involved are *Oestrus ovis*, normally associated with sheep and found everywhere that sheep are kept, and *Rhinoestrus purpureus*, associated with horses and confined to the Old World.

PSEUDOPARASITES

Human beings can be infested with insects which are in a commensal rather than a truly parasitic relationship with them. The phenomenon is well-known in many areas of zoology and frequently is an obligatory mode of life for the commensal species involved. In man infestations with commensal insects always have the character of being both accidental and temporary. In addition certain parasites of animals may have a temporary and accidental relationship with man which never develops to the point of true parasitism.

Hippoboscidae (louse flies)

This Family of Diptera is adapted to a truly parasitic relationship with various birds and mammals, being bloodsucking ectoparasites in fur and feathers. Many species have the wings reduced or absent, the body is flattened, and the legs adapted for grasping hair or feathers. After gaining access to man they cling tenaciously, but not all species will bite. In the United States *Pseudolynchia canariensis*, normally a parasite of swifts, often gives a painful bite, but the cosmopolitan sheep ked *Melophagus ovinus*, a wingless species, rarely does. Bequaert[24] has reviewed their relationships with man.

Collembola (springtails)

Species of this order occasionally infest man, the hair of the head being the usual site, although not the only one. Leclerq[25] suggests that the presence of excess fat on the scalp may contribute to an infestation. Numerous species have been recorded, from clean and dirty persons. No lesions and no ill-effects attend their presence. Infestations may be remarkably heavy and continue for some time, or be transitory and dispersed in a few hours.

Coleoptera (beetles)

Transitory infestations with beetles are recorded, most commonly from the alimentary canal, reminiscent of pseudomyiasis. The beetles are in no sense truly parasitic as they are harmed or killed during passage through the intestines. Both adult and larval forms may affect man, usually by ingestion of infested food, but usually little harm ensues. The mealworm *Tenebrio molitor* is frequently involved, as are the various flour beetles and grain weevils. Theodorides'[26, 27] papers examine the subject.

Lepidoptera (butterflies and moths)

The ingestion of Lepidopterous larvae with uncooked food is called scholechiasis. It must usually pass quite unnoticed for records are rare.

References

1. Ewing, H. E. (1942). The origin and classification of the Apterygota. *Proc. Ent. Soc. Washington*, **44**, 75
2. Metcalfe, Z. P. (1940). How many insects are there in the world? *Ent. News*, **51**, 219
3. Snodgrass, R. E. (1951). *Comparative Studies on the Head of Mandibulate Arthropods*. (New York: Ithaca)
4. Imms, A. D. (1977). *A General Textbook of Entomology* (10th edition). (London: Chapman and Hall)
5. Askew, R. R. (1971). *Parasitic Insects*. (London: Heinemann)
6. Busvine, J. R. (1978). *Insects and Hygiene* (3rd edition in preparation). (London: Methuen)

7. James, M. T. and Harwood, R. F. (1969). *Herms' Medical Entomology* (6th edition). (New York: Macmillan)
8. Ke Chung Kim and Ludwig, H. W. (1978). The family classification of the Anoplura. *Systematic Entomology*, **3**, 249
9. Hopkins, G. H. E. (1949). The host associations of the lice of mammals. *Proc. Zool. Soc. Lond.*, **119**, 387
10. Buxton, P. A. (1947). *The Louse* (2nd edition). (London: Arnold)
11. Maunder, J. W. (1977). Human lice—biology and control. *Roy. Soc. Health J.*, **97**, 29
12. Poisson, R. (1951). Ordre des Hétéroptères. In: Grassé, P. P., *Traité de Zoologie*, **10**, 1657
13. Johnson, C. G. (1942). The ecology of the bed-bug, *Cimex lectularius* in Britain. *J. Hyg.*, **41**, 345
14. Usinger, R. L. (1966). *Monograph of Cimicidae.* (Maryland: Thomas Say Foundation)
15. Usinger, R. L. (1944). The Triatominae of North and Central America and the West Indies and their public health significance. *Publ. Hlth, Bull.*, **288**, 83 pp.
16. Lane, J. (1974). The preservation and mounting of insects of medical importance. World Health Organization WHO/VBC/74.502
17. Smith, K. G. V. (1973). *Insects and Other Arthropods of Medical Importance.* (London: Trustees of the British Museum)
18. Bolam, R. M. and Burtt, E. (1956). *Br. Med. J.*, (i), 1130
19. Zumpt, F. (1965). *Myiasis in Man and Animals in the Old World.* (London: Butterworths)
20. Scott, H. G. (1964). Human myiasis in North America (1952–1962 inclusive). *Fla. Entom.*, **47**, 255
21. Lee, D. J. (1968). Human myiasis in Australia *Med. J. Aust.*, **1**, 170
22. Oldroyd, H. and Smith, K. G. V. (1973). Eggs and larvae of flies. In: Smith, K. G. V. *Insects and Other Arthropods of Medical Importance.* (London: Trustees of the British Museum)
23. West, L. S. (1951). *The Housefly.* (New York: Ithaca)
24. Bequaert, J. (1953). The Hippoboscidae or louse-flies (Diptera) of mammals and birds. *Entomologica Am.* (1952), **32**, 1; (1953) **33**, 211
25. Leclerq, M. (1969). *Entomological Parasitology.* (Oxford: Pergamon)
26. Theodorides, J. (1949). Les Coléoptères parasites accidentels de l'homme. *Ann. Parasit.* (1948), **23**, 348; (1949) **24**, 110
27. Theodorides, J. (1950). The parasitological, medical and veterinary importance of Coleoptera. *Acta Tropica*, **7**, 48

3
Mites and Ticks

R. E. CHURCH

CLASSIFICATION

Mites and ticks belong to the Order Acarina which is one of the seven Orders of the Class Arachnida, one of the largest Classes of the Phylum Arthropoda. Unlike insects, in which the head, thorax and abdomen are easily recognized, in the Acarina signs of segmentation are lost and the cephalothorax—formed by fusion of the head and thorax—is fixed with the abdomen. The anterior segment of the body carries the mouthparts, forming a false head known as the gnathosoma in mites or the capitulum in ticks. The mouthparts consist of palps which are sensory organs, often leglike, and the chelicerae which vary in appearance depending on whether they are used by the species for tearing or piercing. The epistome and hypostome (upper and lower lip) are particularly conspicuous in ticks.

In common with all Arachnids the adult has four pairs of legs consisting of six segments. The genital opening is placed ventrally and there are separate sexes, sexual dimorphism being marked in all but the soft ticks.

The Order Acarina is divided into four Suborders:

1. Ixodides, which contains the hard and soft ticks
2. Mesostigmata, including mites such as *Dermanyssus gallinae* (red poultry mite) and *Ornithonyssus bacoti* (tropical rat mite)
3. Sarcoptiformes includes *Sarcoptes scabiei*
4. Trombidiformes, commonly known as chiggers, harvest mites (*Trombicula autumnalis*) and scrub-itch mites.

GEOGRAPHICAL DISTRIBUTION

Mites and ticks have a worldwide distribution, but the species differ and in many their importance lies in their role as vectors of disease in particular areas.

Sarcoptes scabiei (var. *hominis*) is ubiquitous but even so its frequency has not only varied over the years but also from country to country. Thus Orkin[1] in 1971 surveyed the incidence of scabies around the world and found that it was high in England, France, Poland, West Germany, East Germany, Russia, Portugal, Italy, Morocco, Argentina, Brazil and Mexico. The epidemic had not involved the United States or Canada and the condition was rare in Venezuela, Uruguay, Hungary, Rumania, Japan and Australia. However by 1973–4 there was a general increase in scabies in the United States[2] though by 1975 some dermatologists thought that the peak was passed. Similarly in Spain the epidemic started in 1971, increased in 1973 and appeared to remit in 1975[3]. In other parts of the world such as India and Bangladesh scabies remains a severe problem.

Animal scabies also has its differences in incidence and distribution so that Orkin[1] also noted an increase in canine scabies in the United States since 1963. Cat scabies (*Notoedres cati*) is rare in Britain but in Czechoslovakia and Japan it is more common than mange in dogs.

Other mites having a patchy geographical distribution are the Trombiculae. *T. autumnalis* (the harvest mite) occurs in pockets over most of Northern Europe and in Britain it is particularly prevalent over the chalk downs in south England. Other Trombiculae are of importance in Asia as vectors of scrub typhus and rickettsial infection.

Argasid ticks (or soft ticks) are widely distributed in the tropics and sub-tropics. They are more common in the drier parts of the tropics and in areas where the rainfall is heavy they seek a drier microclimate. Their distribution is patchy as they have a marked host preference, some seeking avian hosts, some mammals, while some species such as *Ornithodorus moubata* live in the cracked walls and floors of mud houses and use man as one of their hosts.

The Ixodidae (hard ticks) have a worldwide distribution and in Britain alone 16 species of hard ticks are recorded of which the commonest is *I. ricinus* (the sheep tick). Owing to its need of a microenvironment of almost saturated air and temperatures which reach 15 °C for long enough for development the tick is most commonly found in areas of woodland and scrub or in woodland and heath covered with a mat of old vegetation. Scotland, the Northern Pennines, Wales and the moors of Devon and Cornwall are therefore its breeding grounds in Britain[4].

In the forests of central Europe the hard tick is so common that road signs give notice of the danger and Ixodides are said to be spreading from their original sites in Russia, via Hungary and Czechoslovakia to Southern Germany and Austria carrying with them the virus of encephalitis[5], though evidence for this spread is disputed.

SCABIES

History

'The Itch' and arguments about its association with mites have a long history. Hebra[6] considered that the Biblical 'Zaraath' could have been scabies and that the cure of Naaman, captain of the host of the King of Syria, by Elisha (Kings, ii. 5.) who advised him to wash seven times in the Jordan was due to the high sulphur content of the water.

The first reference to the acarus of scabies is in a work entitled *Physika* written in the 12th century by Saint Hildegard. She refers to the itch mites as suren, a term which was used until the 18th century.

Cestoni of Leghorn, a pharmacist, and Giovanni Bonomo are generally credited with being the first to describe the acarus as the cause of scabies in a letter written in 1687 and this was the first time the microscope had been used to identify a minute organism as the cause of disease. Their account is so detailed that little can be added today, nevertheless it was soon forgotten only to be recorded in greater detail by Wichmann[7]. Scepticism still persisted however, especially in France where a prize was offered early in the 19th century for anyone who could find an acarus. Eventually in 1834 Renucci at the Hôpital St. Louis, succeeded in teaching the medical men of Paris how to find the acarus and later wrote a thesis on the subject.

The acarus (*Sarcoptes scabiei* var. *hominis*)

The adult female is the form in which the acarus is usually isolated, it is approximately 1/60 of an inch in length—just visible to the naked eye; the male is about half this size. (Figure 3.1). The body of the mite resembles a tortoise, rounded on the back and flat below with a striated white skin. On the ventral surface thickened bars in the cuticle support articulation of the legs. The head has a pair of toothed chelicerae and a pair of short palps. The two pairs of hind legs bear bristles in the female, whereas the male has one bristle and a sucker.

Colonization of a new host is accomplished by a newly-fertilized female. She can travel over the skin at about 2.5 cm per minute and when placed on the skin soon begins to burrow into it using the jaws and the front two pairs of legs for digging. The front legs end in suckers with which the mite anchors itself as it digs with a cutting edge on the terminal joint of the leg, probably using the bristles in the hind legs for leverage. Once in the burrow, spines on the creature's back anchor it in position when necessary. When in the burrow, which can take as little as 15 minutes, the female remains in it for the rest of her life, laying about two eggs daily for one or two months. The eggs are smooth and white measuring about 0.17 × 0.09 mm, they hatch in 3–4 days and the larva emerges (Figure 3.2).

The larva resembles the adult but has only three pairs of legs, the anterior legs bearing suckers and the single pair of posterior legs bristles. They leave the

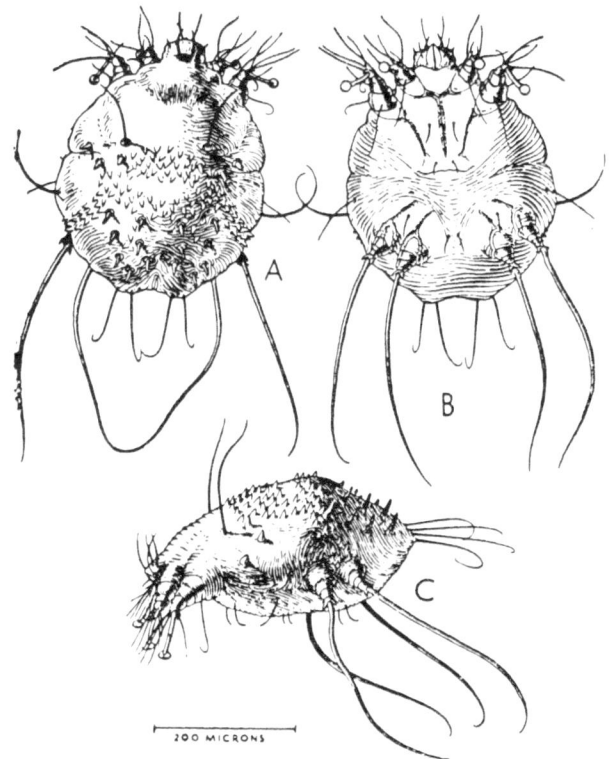

200 MICRONS

Figure 3.1 Adult female of *Sarcoptes scabiei* var. *hominis*. A. Dorsal view; B. Ventral view; C. Lateral view

burrow and shelter in hair follicles for about three days before moulting to form the nymph with four pairs of legs. The nymph moults again, once to form the adult male or twice before becoming the adult female.

Adult males also burrow into the skin but only make short burrows which they leave to seek the female. Copulation takes place by the male facing in the opposite direction to the female and resting his ventral surface containing his sexual organ over the dorsal copulatory orifice of the female. The male mates once only and about two days after copulation the female begins to lay eggs through an oviduct leading to a pore on the ventral surface of the body. The whole cycle from egg to ovigerous female takes about 14 days, but although a high proportion of the eggs hatch, only about 10% of mites reach maturity.

Transmission

The acarus can move quite swiftly, over a glass slide for example, at temperatures above 20 °C but below this temperature little movement occurs

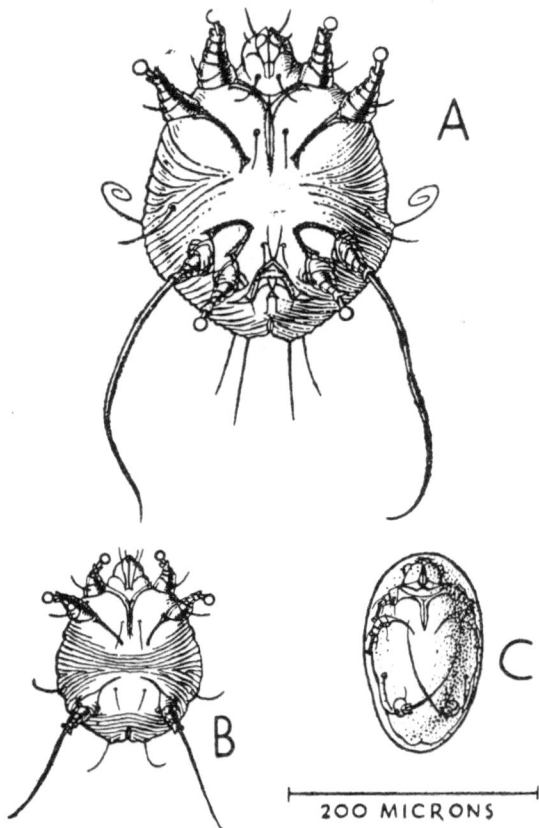

200 MICRONS

Figure 3.2   Stages in the life history of Sarcoptes A. Adult male; B. Larva; C. Egg containing developing embryo

and only in moist conditions does it remain alive for more than a day or two. The likelihood of indirect infestation via fomites is therefore remote; direct and prolonged person to person contact is usually necessary for spread of the disease. Mellanby[8] carried out numerous experiments during the Second World War to determine whether bedding and clothes could carry the infestation and was unable to demonstrate that they could. The scales shed by patients with Norwegian scabies do contain numerous mites which can be recovered from room dust and these might be responsible for some of the rapid spread of infestation from these cases.

The course of the disease

Experimentally induced infestations have given the most accurate picture of the disease. Infestation by a single ovigerous female is followed by a second generation of adult females in three to four weeks. During that time the subject is symptom-free. During the next two months there is rapid growth in the mite population and about the beginning of this period the host becomes sensitized. A widespread, very itchy, papular eruption results, scratching and sepsis destroys many of the mites and the disease then settles to a chronic itchy eruption in which the number of mites carried is on average only about twelve.

Reinfestation in a previously infested and sensitized individual causes a severe reaction with intense itching round the burrow of the ovigerous female so that the mites are usually rapidly removed by scratching. Even if not, the mite colony remains small in number and may eventually die out. There is therefore a partial immunity due to antibody function. Immunological measurements in patients with scabies of under three weeks' duration and longer durations showed raised IgG and IgM in both groups, implying a humoral response to scabies, though secondary bacterial infection could also play some part[9].

Symptoms and signs

Intense itching especially when warm in bed at night is the patient's main complaint; occasionally secondary sepsis may become so severe that boils and impetigo overshadow the itch. The story of others in the family or friends itching increases the probability of scabies as the diagnosis.

Itching commences at the time of development of the sensitization eruption which usually becomes widespread and affects the elbows, axillary folds and buttocks in particular, producing non-specific scratched papules which are also disseminated over the rest of the body but sparing the face. The diagnostic lesions are burrows which may be few in number and hard to find (Figure 3.3). Their sites of election are the sides of the fingers and finger webs, the ulnar border of the palms, the flexor aspect of the wrists and the soles. It has been suggested[10] that the acarus avoids areas containing dense hair follicles. Occasionally burrows can be found in other areas especially in infants in whom they may even appear on the face and scalp. These burrows Madsen[11] demonstrated in crusts rather than in the horny layer. Small tense vesicles often occur on the palms and soles as part of the sensitization phenomenon and are not to be confused with burrows.

The burrows consist of wavy slightly black lines several millimetres long in the epidermis, often with a mild inflammatory erythema around them. At the more intact end of the burrow the acarus can be seen as a black dot just visible to the naked eye. In some, especially children, whose reaction is severe, the burrow may become vesicular and hide the acarus.

In infants scattered pink nodules 0.5–1.0 cm across, usually on the trunk and resembling 'blind boils', may be the predominating feature (Figure 3.4). Similar lesions commonly affect the penis and scrotum in adults and are so characteristic that they clinch the diagnosis. Occasionally nodules may appear on the trunk in adults and it is common for them to persist and remain itchy after treatment[12].

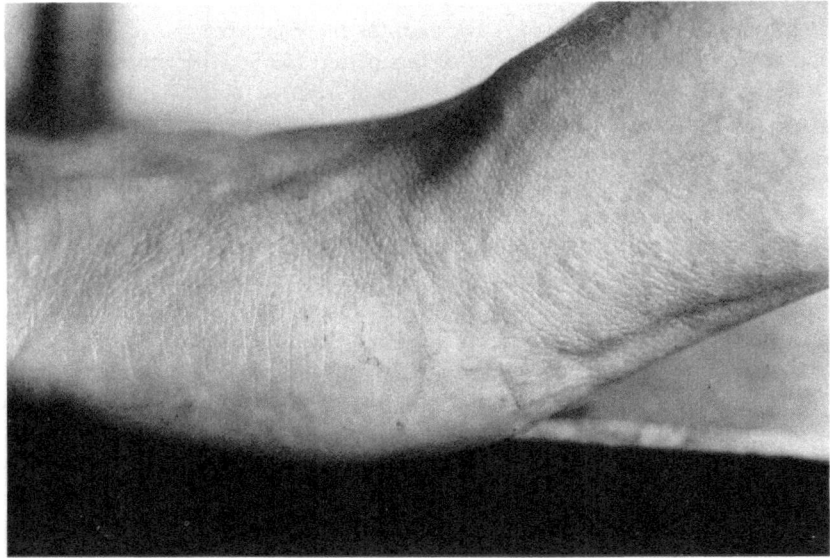

Figure 3.3   Scabies burrows

Histological examination of such nodules reveals a dense pleomorphic infiltrate simulating a reticulosis[13]. An acarus could only be found in one of the six specimens examined and it remained in the horny layer of the epidermis.

Occasionally the sensitization eruption resembles papular urticaria, a diagnosis which should be made with caution in the middle of a scabies epidemic.

Diagnosis

The diagnosis is confirmed by isolating an acarus and demonstrating it under the microscope (Figure 3.5). Without this the diagnosis is often heard with resentment and disbelief by the patient. With the aid of a spotlight and a watchmaker's lens a search should be made for a typical active burrow, starting on the hands and wrists where 70% of burrows are found[14]; if unsuccessful elbows, feet and external genitalia in the male should be examined. Taking a burrow in which an acarus can clearly be seen the horny layer is broken with a pin and the acarus, then visible as a shiny white speck, can be induced to adhere to the pin and transferred to a microscope slide. A ring of ink round it helps to position it under the microscope objective. In black skins it is not so easy to spot the acarus, in which case the burrow can be scraped with a curette and the curettings mounted in 10% potash under a coverslip.

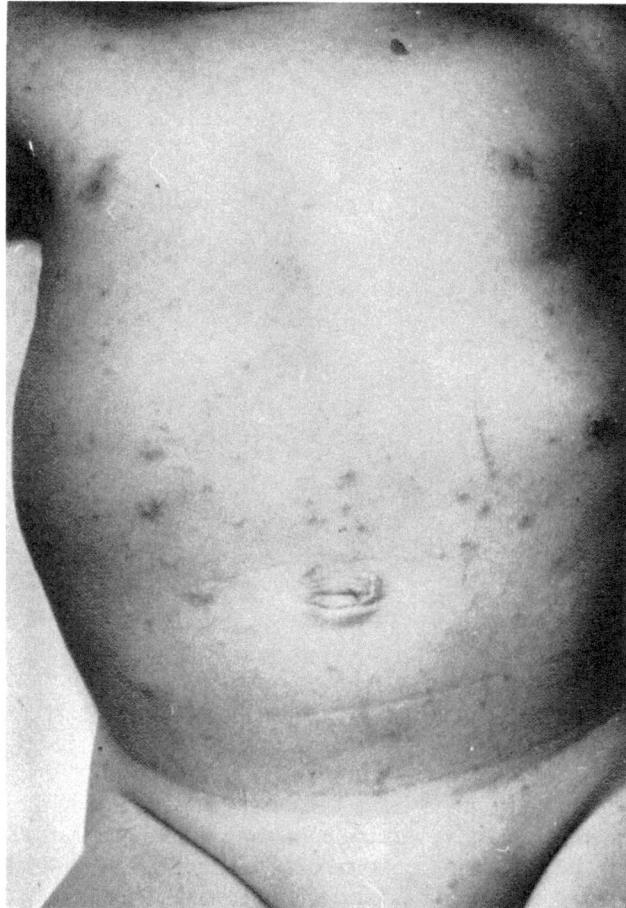

Figure 3.4 Scabies in an infant

Complications

Sepsis is especially likely in those whose general hygiene is poor. Vesicles become pustules and lesions of impetigo, ecthyma and furunculosis cause more discomfort than the itch. If secondary infection with haemolytic streptococci occurs acute glomerulonephritis may result. An epidemic of scabies associated with glomerulonephritis was reported from Trinidad[15] but such an association is very rare in non-tropical climates[16].

Norwegian scabies or crusted scabies was first described in a leper by Boeck. Peripheral or cortical loss of sensation may be responsible for some of the cases seen in mongols and those with senile dementia etc. but impaired cell-

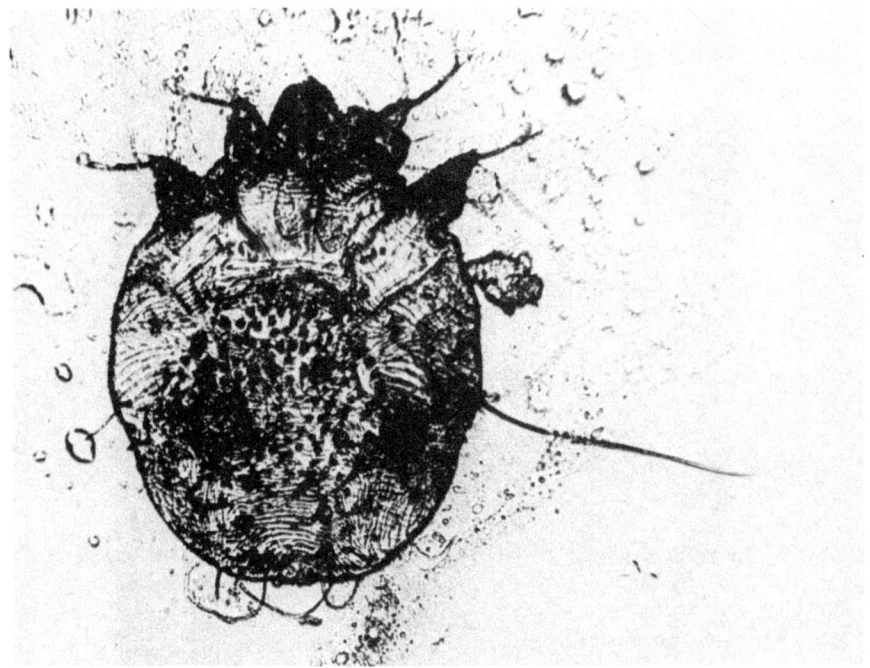

Figure 3.5 *Sarcoptes scabiei*

mediated immunity also plays some part as is demonstrated in the occurrence of the disease in renal transplant patients being treated with azathioprine and prednisolone[17,18]. In such patients the skin lesions become so thick and scaly that they mimic psoriasis; this is particularly so round the fingers, finger nails, palms and soles. Eventually the whole skin may be affected to produce a picture resembling exfoliative dermatitis. In a biopsy the histology of the thickened horny layer resembles Gruyère cheese, its many holes each containing an acarus. The manifestations are so unlike ordinary scabies that the diagnosis is often overlooked until several of those nursing the patient develop the disease[19].

Treatment

Benzyl benzoate lotion is still the time-honoured treatment of scabies in adults and there is no convincing evidence that the acarus has become resistant to it as has been suggested. Benzyl benzoate stings when applied to children's skin and in affected families with children 'Tetmosol' (monosulfiram) can be used. This is diluted with two or three parts of water before each application and adults should be warned to avoid alcohol before and during its use (its effects are similar to ingested disulfiram—'Antabuse'). There are several other anti-scabetics on the market. After one application of benzyl benzoate by a trained nurse live acari cannot be recovered from a patient; however, human fallibility being what it is, the following regime is recommended. The patient takes a bath, scrubbing the fingers and hands gently with a soft nailbrush, dries the skin then applies the antiscabetic lotion with a paintbrush to every area of the skin below the neck, paying particular attention to hands and soles. The lotion is allowed to dry and the previously worn clothes resumed. On the second day the same process is repeated, clean clothes worn and clean sheets put on the bed. No special attention need be given to the clothes or bedclothes other than ordinary washing. It is vital to stress that every member of the household, whether itching or not, must be treated otherwise early symptom-free carriers may reintroduce the infestation.

The patient must also be warned against repeated application of the anti-scabetic lotion even though the itching may settle down slowly, otherwise it can cause dermatitis. Any post-treatment itch can be treated with calamine lotion or a dilute steroid cream. Nodules which persist after treatment may respond to the application of Eurax ointment (Crotamiton) twice daily; if not they can, where suitable, be injected with hydrocortisone acetate solution BP. If sepsis is present the scabies should be treated first and when the course is finished an appropriate antibiotic cream applied unless streptococcal infection is also present, in which case systemic penicillin should be given without delay.

In problem families in which scabies is difficult to eradicate it is best to arrange for the household to be treated at the local disinfestation centre which exists in most cities.

Epidemiology

For a disease which is spread only by close personal contact and which can be cured so rapidly and easily, scabies has proved remarkably difficult to eradicate. Its epidemics have been the subject of comment for the past 200 years and optimism at times of its disappearance has proved ill-founded. Writing in 1766 William Buchan stated, 'The itch is now by cleanliness banished from every genteel family in Britain. It still however prevails among the poorer sort of peasants in Scotland and amongst the manufacturers in England'[20]. The situation has not changed.

During the present century there have been three epidemics, the first occurring during the 1914–18 war. The second had already begun before the Second World War[21] and reached its height about 1943. Ten years later scabies had again become very uncommon but from 1957 in England there was a steady increase in the numbers referred to hospitals in cities such as Sheffield and London[22, 23]. The fluctuations of the disease appear in cycles, approximately 15 years of widespread disease being followed by a similar period in which it becomes rare. The reservoirs of disease during its quiescent periods are difficult to establish but it is known that many cases of Norwegian scabies are undiagnosed for long periods and can be the source of localized outbreaks[24]. Small closed communities such as fishermen in Kiel[25] can keep the disease grumbling on in a chronic state and it is not uncommon to see elderly persons living alone who apparently genuinely lead solitary lives and who appear to have suffered from scabies for a very long time.

There have been numerous explanations for the cyclical outbreaks, the most popular of which is the development of herd resistance. It has been pointed out that second attacks of scabies are resisted in the sensitized individual. The theory is that when the level of susceptible subjects reaches a certain threshold the mite population can spread in epidemic proportions[8]. Another factor which plays some part in delaying control of spread is the lack of awareness of the disease by general practitioners trained during its slumps[26,27]. Also the ubiquitous use of local corticosteroids not only delays correct treatment but promotes the spread of disease in the patient[28].

Other explanations have their advocates; poverty and poor hygiene, while still with us, have certainly diminished, sexual promiscuity could be responsible for some of the spread, but figures culled from VD clinic attendances are biased and scabies has been shown to be predominantly a disease of families and young children just as canine scabies is a disease of puppies[8,29]. A survey of an Indian village[30] showed that 6% of the total population and 20% of households had scabies. Eighty-one per cent of those infested were under the age of 14 and there was a significant correlation between limitation of sleeping space and prevalence of disease. Increased travel and movements of populations could also play some part. Finally we may be concentrating on the soil when we should be studying the seed; Orkin[1] noted that there had been a marked increase in canine scabies in the United States since 1963. Sudden mutation to allow the canine mite to adapt to man seems unlikely but since 1971 human scabies has reached epidemic proportions in the United States and it seems possible that explosions in mite population of both kinds could be the cause rather than the result of the disease spread.

Control in the community

When scabies became uncommon after the Second World War it ceased to be notifiable is most areas of Britain. As the incidence increased attempts were made to control it by a system of voluntary notification and a follow-up scheme by health visitors[22]. The number of cases continued to increase in subsequent years so that in Sheffield in 1972–3, 1482 cases were traced in 609 households[31] and it appeared that this was only the tip of the iceberg. In 1975 the Sheffield Area Health Authority made scabies a notifiable disease but despite a follow-up scheme the numbers notified each year since have remained constant. In a smaller community eradication is possible; Kanaaneh[32] dealt with an outbreak of scabies in an Arab village with a population of 3000, 22%

of which had scabies. A team of eight nurses, one male nurse, a sanitary inspector and a health educator spent three months collecting data, two months on an information campaign and one week in treatment. During the follow-up period of one year, only one case of scabies occurred, and was treated. This amount of activity is unlikely to be devoted to scabies in the large cities of the Western world but undoubtedly more could be done to bring the disease under control.

MANGE MITES

Sarcoptes scabiei causes sarcoptic mange in dogs; the mites are identical to those which infest humans but are physiologically adapted to a different host and remain host-specific. Experimental attempts to establish the canine mite on human skin caused some scaling and papule formation but mites had disappeared within twelve days[33].

In the dog, usually a young dog[34], the elbow and external ear are the main habitats of the mite though it can affect the whole skin. The affected areas become erythematous, papular, scaly and crusted and hair is lost. The diagnosis is confirmed by examining skin scrapings or by biopsy, when mites can be seen in pockets in the epidermis. Humans in contact with the dog develop tiny crusted papules but no burrows, the lesions being commonest on the arms, round the waist and on the lower legs. Usually more than one person in a household is affected and since it is calculated that about 1% of the 5 million dogs in the United Kingdom has sarcoptic mange[35] the number of cases in humans must be significant.

Notoedres cati is very similar in form to *Sarcoptes* but slightly smaller. it produces mange in cats and results in dry crusted and scaly lesions on the edges of the ears and face; eventually the skin on those areas becomes thickened and leathery. In Great Britain cat scabies is very rare though it has been recorded as the cause of a papular skin eruption[36] but in other countries cat scabies affects man more often than dog scabies.

CHEYLETIELLA INFESTATIONS

'Walking dandruff' is a veterinary name for this infestation of the hair coat of the dog or cat. *C. yasguri* spends its entire life cycle within the hair coat of the host, commonly affecting puppies in which it is found on the nose and head and along the spine and rump. The animal itches and scales of dandruff appear in the affected areas. The eggs of the mite are attached to the hair shafts by short threads, these hatch in a few days and after three moults the life cycle is completed in 34 days[37]. The mites are just visible to the naked eye and microscopic examination of skin scrapings from the animal reveals that the mites have four pairs of legs, bearing combs instead of claws and the accessory mouthparts end in prominent hooks.

C. parasitovax mainly affects cats and rabbits and the distribution of the infestation is more generalized throughout the hair coat. Minor morphological differences occur in the species *yasguri* and *parasitovax*[38] but neither has extreme host specificity and can be found in dogs, cats and rabbits.

Cheyletiella species affect man and are prone to do so when the infested animal is in close contact with its keeper as lapdogs may be. *Cheyletiella* species penetrate the clothing and produce lesions which vary from tiny erythematous macules and papules to vesicular and pustular lesions which leave necrotic crusts after rupture. The sites of predilection are the arms, neck and trunk, especially round the waist. The lesions may be discretely scattered or arranged in groups and as they resolve in about three weeks, they leave pigmentation which may last three to six months. The lesions may therefore be mistaken for eczema or dermatitis herpetiformis[39]. Skin lesions in the human cease when the infestation in the animal has been successfully eradicated but this must include disinfestation of the animal's bedding, soft furnishings in the house and carpets.

BLOOD SUCKING MITES

The red poultry mite (*Dermanyssus gallinae*)

This mite is a common parasite of wild birds such as sparrows, starlings and pigeons but it also attacks poultry and dogs. The nymphs and adults usually feed at night and remain hidden in crevices during the day where they can survive for months without a blood meal. The mites lay their eggs in birds' nests or poultry houses and on hatching produce a six-legged larva which then moults to produce the eight-legged first stage nymph followed by the second stage nymph and adult.

Workers on poultry farms or poultry markets when handling mite-infested poultry are accustomed to bites but more puzzling are those cases in which the mites invade the bedroom from pigeons' nests under the eaves[40] or even the living room from the pet canary[41].

Tropical rat mite (*Ornithonysus bacoti*)

Human cutaneous disease as the result of infestation with this mite is well known in North America[42] but outbreaks have been recorded in England[43] as well as other parts of the world.

The mites are yellow and become red after a blood feed; they measure 0.75 to 1.40 mm and the rodent is their preferred host. The life cycle is in five stages, the egg, the larva, which has three pairs of legs, and the protonymph, deutonymph and adult, all of which have four pairs of legs. The adult can survive eight or nine weeks without feeding and can therefore remain viable for several weeks after extermination of a rat colony, during which time it may travel several hundred feet in search of food. In the human it produces an itchy papular eruption often situated over the shoulders, breasts and arms. If the mite can be found on the patient and identified, a search for rats' nests in attics or furniture should be successful. The mite has been shown to transmit murine typhus, rickettsial pox and tularaemia to other animals but it is of doubtful importance as a vector of human disease.

THE HARVEST MITE (*Trombicula autumnalis*) OR CHIGGER

These mites are bright red or orange in colour, have a velvety appearance due to a bristle coat and have a figure-of-eight shape. They occur over most of

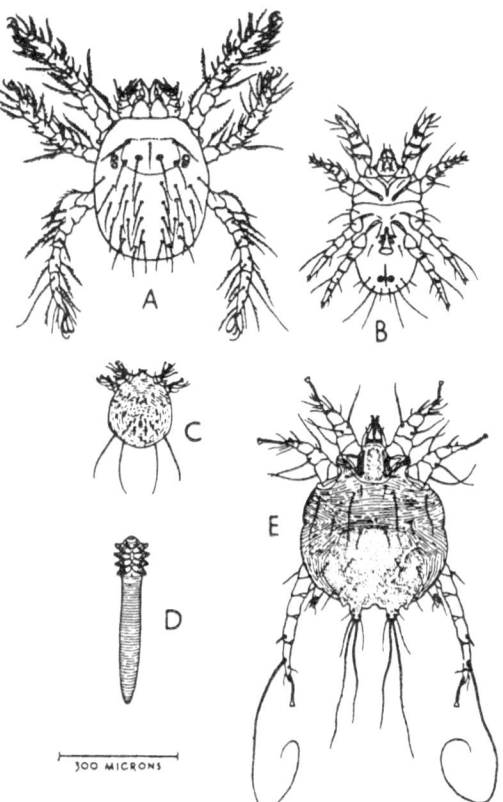

300 MICRONS

Figure 3.6 Mites of medical and veterinary importance: A. *Trombicula autumnalis*; B. *Tyroglyphid*; C. *Notoedrus*; D. *Demodex*; E. *Psoroptes* (sheep mange)

Figures 3.1, 3.2 and 3.6 are reproduced from *Scabies* (1972) by K. Mellanby, (E. W. Classey Ltd., Hampton) by kind permission of author and publishers. Figures 3.3 and 3.5 are from *Practical Dermatology*, 3rd edition (1976) by I. B. Sneddon and R. E. Church (Edward Arnold, London) by kind permission of the publishers.

Northern Europe and in Britain are prolific over the chalk downs, their peak of activity being in September. Other species of *Trombicula* are found throughout the world.

The eggs are laid in the soil and hatch to produce a six-legged larva. The larvae feed on vegetation but require animal protein for further development and it is only at this stage that the mite is parasitic. The larvae climb to the tips of grass blades or of leaves and attach themselves to an animal—commonly rodent or rabbit. On man they crawl up until they reach the constriction of clothing then attach themselves. The mites' salivary excretion digests the skin to form a tube with a hardened wall, the stylostome, which may penetrate the dermis, through which the mite sucks lymph.

Eventually the larvae drop off onto the soil and moult to form the eight-legged nymph which again moults to form the adult. The response of the host to the larva bite depends on the state of allergy. The non-allergic host reacts only with tiny red macules at the sites of bites. In the sensitized human weals, papules and vesicles form which may be accompanied by lymphadenopathy and even a mild febrile illness, the eruption being known as 'scrub itch'. In Eastern Asia *T. akamushi* and *T. deliensis* are vectors of the rickettsia of scrub typhus.

GRAIN MITES (*Pyemotes ventriculosus*)

These mites' chief hosts are the larvae of the grain moth and the wheat jointworm. The female is viviparous and the young emerge in a state of maturity. They occur throughout the world and are the cause of outbreaks of dermatitis among those handling grain, straw and tobacco, thus dockers, millers, farmers and bakers are prone to attack. The mites cause an irritation of human skin to which they attach themselves very loosely so that the reaction may be mainly allergic. Urticarial papules and vesicles are produced especially on the hands, arms and chest. It has been known for the mites to be carried to their homes by workers exposed to them so that other members of their family may develop the skin eruption. Once contact with infested materials ceases the rash swiftly resolves.

HAIR FOLLICLE MITES (*Demodex folliculorum*)

This is a worm-like acarus about 0.3 to 0.4 mm long; it has a rounded head, a thorax from which four pairs of rudimentary legs project and a transversely segmental abdomen with characteristically rounded caudal tip. It is a natural inhabitant of the pilosebaceous follicles in the areas of greatest sebaceous secretion around the face, neck and shoulders. Positioned with its head directed inward, there may be as many as a dozen in the same follicle[44] and they can be found in the debris of expressed comedones. The female having been been fertilized at the follicular orifice lays her eggs in the sebaceous gland. These hatch and the usual two nymphal stages last about a week while the adult has a life of about two weeks. A second species *Demodex brevis* inhabits the sebaceous glands but the significance of this has yet to be worked out.

Demodectic mange

A similar mite *Demodex canis* is part of the normal fauna in even healthy dogs but it is thought that an immunodeficiency state allows massive increase in numbers of the mites causing mange or demodicosis. It is seen almost exclusively in young dogs and there appears to be an hereditary predisposition as well as a tendency for the disease to attack certain breeds such as beagles. The disease may be localized and give rise to several scaly patches of alopecia but may become generalized, secondarily infected and can even be fatal[45].

Pityriasis folliculorum (*Demodex*)

This was first described by Ayres[46] as a diffuse erythema of the face with a nutmeg grater appearance and follicular scaling accompanied by a sensation of itching and burning. It was found in older women who used creams on their face instead of washing. A second type of eruption resembled rosacea in the presence of papules and papulo-pustules.

Microscopic examination of the follicular scales examined in potassium hydroxide revealed large numbers of *Demodex* and the eruption responded rapidly to the application of sulphur ointment. Blepharitis has also been ascribed to the same organism[47].

The number of parasites in follicles in areas of rosacea are increased. It seems possible that this is merely because conditions are suitable for multiplication of the mite rather than its having any pathogenic role in rosacea, however it is postulated that once the level of infestation exceeds a certain threshold an inflammatory reaction is provoked which gives rise to some of the signs of rosacea[48].

FOOD MITES (TYROGLYPHIDS)

A hand lens is sufficient to demonstrate that cheese may contain mites but similar species of mite can be found in many stored foods[49]. Those whose work entails carrying such articles as cheese, bacon, dried figs and flour may develop an itchy papulo-pustular erythema on the areas in contact, principally the forearms and chest. The role of the mite in production of the eruption is debatable as it is unlikely that they bite the skin and it seems to be an allergic type of reaction as dead mites in sufficient numbers can cause the rash. Such outbreaks have been sufficiently common in the past for popular names to be ascribed such as 'grocer's itch' caused by *Glycyphagus domesticus* which was at one time found on poor quality sugar; 'vanillism' due to *Tyrophagus casei* on vanilla pods and 'baker's itch' due to *Tyrophagus farinae*. The dermatitis caused by stored food mites heals rapidly when contact with infested food ceases. (Mites are also discussed in Chapters 8 and 9.)

TICKS

Ticks are larger than mites and are bloodsucking parasites at all stages. Most are not host-specific which makes them of importance as disease vectors. There are two kinds of tick, the soft (Argasidae) ticks and the hard tick (Ixodidae). Argasidae ticks are mainly found in warmer climates as parasites of birds and in Britain only the Ixodidae are important as parasites of wild animals which can attach themselves to domestic animals and man.

Hard ticks (Ixodidae)

Hard ticks have a hard shield shaped plate (scutum) which covers the dorsum in the male and only the anterior part of the dorsum of the female, whose body can distend greatly on feeding. There are 16 genera of Ixodidae and they can be differentiated by differences in the capitulum which projects in front of the body and is visible from above. In Britain the commonest is the sheep tick (*Ixodes ricinus* or castor bean tick) which transmits the louping ill in sheep. *Rhipicephalus sanguineus* is a parasite of dogs and can reproduce easily in buildings, unlike most other species which inhabit grass and undergrowth, as although each stage of development can exist for months without a meal they are very sensitive to temperature and humidity. This means that in temperate climates their activity is seasonal, being dormant in winter, seeking to feed in spring and autumn and undergoing development in the warmth of the summer, during which time parasitism rarely takes place.

The female tick having attached itself to its host may feed for over a week, in which time it swells to the size of a pea. It is a pool feeder, cutting skin and capillaries with the mouthpiece and feeding on the extravasated blood, returning the excess of water and ions to the host via its salivary glands. Having completed the meal the female drops off onto the ground and lays her eggs in a single large brown mass covered with a viscous secretion to prevent desiccation. After 2–7 weeks each hatches as a six-legged larva or seed tick. After about 5 days' rest this climbs to the tips of leaves or grass, clinging by the hind legs and waiting to seize a passing animal. Having fed for some days on this it drops off to hide and rest for up to three months until it moults to form the eight-legged nymph. After a few days this repeats the process of seeking a host by climbing to the tips of foliage; when successful it feeds again for about a week and again drops off to spend some weeks resting before the final moult produces the adult. The adult male's task is then to mate with a female, and while the male may take a short blood meal it is the female who attaches for days to gorge herself with blood. The adult can live for up to 19 months and although the life cycle is usually completed in a year, such is the tick's ability to survive unfed that the cycle may take two or three years. (See also Chapter 9.)

Soft ticks (Argasidae)

Soft ticks have a rough cuticle folded into creases and there is no dorsal plate, the sexes are similar and the capitulum is not visible from above. They differ from hard ticks in that they are rapid and nocturnal feeders and at each stage of development may feed on several different hosts which increases their potential as disease vectors.

Although they are mainly parasites of birds, in regions where they are endemic they attack all kinds of animals. The poultry tick and the pigeon tick may bite man and the spinous ear tick (*Otobius megnini*) which is a parasite of many domestic animals, including dogs and cats, will often bite man. The ear tick is found in the southern United States; the larvae and nymphs infest the external ear of the host causing severe irritation which makes the animal shake its head vigorously and scratch the ear. The adults live in outbuildings, walls etc., and as they can survive for up to a year without a meal it may be necessary to spray buildings with malathion to eradicate them.

Tick bites in man

Ticks feed through a single tube which conveys blood inwards and the saliva outwards[50]. As well as conveying excess of water and ions back to the host, histamine, anticoagulants and other toxic substances are injected from the salivary glands. The reaction round the site of tick bites is often severe causing a large annular area of wealing. Bites of the soft ticks of the genus *Argus* which includes pigeon and fowl ticks are especially severe. As they feed briefly the tick may not be seen and the area of the bite may develop an Arthus-like reaction resulting in an area of necrosis.

TOXIC REACTIONS TO TICK BITES

Hard ticks remain attached for long periods and there may be little reaction and no discomfort from the bite so that its engorged body is the first thing noticed by the human host[51].

The severe reaction to the bite of the soft tick *Ornithodorus tholozani* is seen in Israel and known as ornithodoriasis. Multiple nodules with haemorrhagic punctum wounds develop causing intense pruritus. The lesions begin to subside after 12 days and heal leaving pigmentation[52].

A persistent granulomatous reaction at the site of tick bites can be a foreign body reaction to retained mouthparts, but as excision of the bite has been shown to be ineffective in preventing granuloma formation[53] it could be due to a chronic immunological reaction. Alopecia may appear within a week around tick bites in the scalp, forming a bald patch about 3–4 cm across. It is presumed to be due to toxins and regrowth of hair is rapid[54].

European farmers exposed to numerous tick bites in the harvest time suffer general malaise, urticaria and vomiting known as ixodism. Salivary toxins are presumed responsible and could be the cause of some of the cases of tick bite pyrexia described in North America.

Tick paralysis

The Rocky Mountain wood tick (*Dermacentor andersoni*), a hard tick, was the cause of 93 cases of tick paralysis in British Columbia between 1928 and 1968[55] of which 12 cases were fatal. Other species have caused similar paralysis in other parts of the world including members of the genus *Ixodes* in Australia, Europe and South Africa. Individual ticks of the same species vary in their toxin production which is in some way associated with egg production[45].

Children are affected five times more commonly than adults and in 70% of cases of paralysis the tick is attached to the head or neck where it may be hidden under the hair. Such a position also seems to make the toxin more virulent. After the bite there is a latent period of five days during which the victim may merely become irritable, then over a period of about 24 hours or even less[56] an ascending flaccid paralysis develops which can be fatal if it involves the respiratory centres. There is usually no pain, no fever and the white blood cell count and cerebrospinal fluid remain normal. It appears to be caused by a neurotoxin secreted by the tick's salivary glands and recovery is remarkably swift once the tick is discovered and removed.

INFECTIONS TRANSMITTED BY TICKS

Erythema chronicum migrans

This type of annular erythema starts in exposed areas of the skin and may expand greatly. In Sweden 77 patients were treated at the Karolinska Hospital between 1948 and 1957 and 27% gave a history of a tick bite. The condition responded to massive doses of penicillin[57]. Degos[58] found positive micro-agglutination tests for rickettsiae in six out of seven cases and successfully treated them with broad spectrum antibiotics.

Acrodermatitis atrophicans

This condition occurs in a belt running through northern, central and eastern Europe in areas where *Ixodes ricinus* is common. Successful inoculation of human volunteers and the fact that the early stages respond to penicillin therapy imply an infective agent and it is suggested that it might be conveyed by tick bites. It could be related to *erythema chronicum migrans* which its early lesions resemble. Single or multiple red nodules or plaques develop on the limbs and may extend to the trunk. They extend over months or years to form annular lesions, the centre of which becomes atrophic, smooth, hairless and poikilodermatous.

Relapsing fever

Dutton demonstrated in 1901 that the soft tick *Ornithodorus moubata* was the vector of relapsing fever in Central Africa and the spirochaete which it carries was named after him. Unlike the lice-borne disease which occurs in epidemics, the tick-transmitted disease is endemic and usually sporadic. Another area where the disease is endemic extends round the shores of the Mediterranean through Arabia to Kashmir. The Mediterranean type is caused by *Spirochaeta hispanica* and transmitted by *Ornithodorus erraticus*. In a third endemic area in central and western USA the spirochaetes have a remarkable specificity for their vectors after which they are named (*O. turicatae, O. parkeri* and *O. hermsii*)[59].

Infection in man is commonly acquired from injected saliva but the manner of transmission varies according to the stage of development of the tick. In the case of *O. moubata* in the adult stage, the coxal fluid contains large numbers of spirochaetes and there is therefore risk of infection even by handling the tick, particularly if it is crushed. In the case of *T. duttoni* infection the tick ovaries are invaded and the infection may thus be transmitted congenitally through at least three generations of ticks.

Relapsing fever has an incubation period of about a week and starts abruptly with fever, headache, joint and muscle pains, photophobia and bronchitis. The temperature reaches 40 to 40.5 °C, there may be an erythematous rash and later rose spots on the trunk and limbs. The initial attack lasts two to eight days and if untreated is followed by a remission of several days then a less severe relapse. The disease responds to treatment with chlortetracycline or high doses of penicillin.

Rickettsial infections

Rocky Mountain spotted fever is the most serious of the tick-borne rickettsioses. It was the first to be studied by Ricketts in 1906 after whom the organism is named and who showed that the Ixodid tick *Dermacentor andersoni* was the vector. This type of spotted fever has an incubation period of a week after the bite and is characterized by high fever, muscle and joint pains and a widespread rash appearing about the sixth day. Some cases may be fatal.

Unlike louse-borne typhus the cases are sporadic. The reservoir of infection is in animals and the infection can be transmitted to man by ticks at all stages of development or even from contamination with tick faeces or body fluid. Transmission between humans or even back to ticks does not occur. The disease, usually milder in form, occurs in many other parts of the world and changes its name according to place. Thus in South America it is known as São Paulo typhus, in Australia Queensland typhus, Fièvre Boutonneuse, Indian tick typhus etc. There are several hard ticks known to be vectors the commonest being *Rhipicephalus sanguineus* and *Haemaphysalis leachi*—both dog ticks.

Q fever was first recognized in Queensland but has since been reported in America, round the Mediterranean and Europe including Britain and many other parts of the world. The infection is carried by sheep, goats, cattle and birds. The organism, *Rickettsia burneti* is transmitted to man on occasions by tick bites, in Britain by *Ixodes ricinus*, but more often infection is acquired through ingestion of infected meat or handling infected animals. The illness is usually mild and consists of fever, headache and occasionally pneumonitis lasting from a few days to about a fortnight.

Virus infections

Tick-borne virus infections are most prevalent in Central Europe and Russia. The group B viruses involved include the only British tick-borne virus which causes louping ill in sheep but which can affect man[60], and in Russia a spring–summer encephalitis and Omsk haemorrhagic fever. In Central Europe tick-borne encephalitis follows the bites of various ticks of which *Ixodes persulcatus* and *Ixodes ricinus* are the most important. The areas mainly involved are Hungary, Czechoslovakia, Austria and Southern Germany, 1000 cases of encephalitis being recorded each year caused by tick bites[5]. A considerable percentage of lymphocytic meningitis cases can be shown by antibody tests to be tick-borne encephalitis. A high ESR and high white blood cell count are characteristic. Harasek[61] described 38 cases in children, in two of whom myelitis with flaccid paresis of the upper limbs developed. All the cases recovered without persistent injury to brain or muscles. No specific therapy is known.

Group A virus causes Crimean haemorrhagic fever and the well-known Colorado tick fever. The latter has been shown to be transmitted by *Dermacentor andersoni* and its animal hosts are ground squirrels, chipmunks and deer mice.

Tularaemia

This disease caused by the bacillus *Pasteurelia tularensis* is primarily a disease of wild rodents. Infection is usually acquired by direct contact with infected carcasses but it is sometimes conveyed to man by Ixodid ticks.

REMOVING TICKS

The mouthparts of ticks are securely embedded in the skin and will remain behind if the tick is just wrenched off. Various methods of inducing the tick to release its hold are advocated and that most readily available is the hot end of a matchstick. Alternatives are dabbing with ether or petrol or suffocating the tick with a generous covering of soft paraffin.

Outbreaks of tick infestation in kennels or stables may necessitate spraying the woodwork and crevices with an insecticide spray.

References

1. Orkin, M. (1971). Resurgence of Scabies. *J. Am. Med. Assoc.*, **217**, 593
2. Shaw, P. K. and Juranek, D. D. (1976). Recent trends in scabies in the United States. *J. Infect. Dis.*, **134**, 414
3. Aza, A. B. and Alvarez, R. M. (1976). Escabiosis incidentia y consideraciones epidemiologicas en la region Asturiana. *Rev. San. Sig. Pub.*, **50**, 929
4. Macleod, J. (1962). Ticks and disease in domestic stock in Great Britain. In D. R. Arthur (ed.) *Aspects of Disease Transmission by Ticks* (London. Zoological Soc.) p. 29.
5. Ronay, G. (1977). Deadly tick on westward march. *The Times*, 14.11.77
6. Hebra, F. (1868). *On Diseases of the Skin*, **2**, 164 (London: New Sydenham Society)
7. Wichmann, J. E. (1786). *Aetiologie Der Kratze.* (Hanover)
8. Mellanby, K. (1943). *Scabies.* (London. Oxford Univ. Press)
9. Hancock, B. W. and Ward, A. N. (1974). Serum immunoglobulins in scabies. *J. Invest. Dermatol.*, **63**, 482
10. Madsen, A. (1965). Why *Acarus scabiei* avoids the face. *Acta Dermato-Venereol.*, **45**, 167
11. Madsen, A. (1970). Mite burrows in crusts from young infants. *Acta Dermato-Venereol.*, **50**, 391
12. Ayres, S. Jr. and Anderson, N. P. (1932). Persistent nodules in scabies, histological observations and treatment. *Arch. Derm. Syph.*, **25**, 485
13. Thomson, J., Cochrane, T., Cochran, R. and McQueen, A. (1974). Histology simulating reticulosis in persistent nodular scabies. *Br. J. Dermatol.*, **90**, 421
14. Bartley, W. and Mellanby, K. (1944). The parasitology of human scabies (women and children). *Parasitology*, **35**, 207
15. Swartman, M., Potter, E. V., Finkler, J. F., Poon-King, T. and Earle, D. P. (1972). Epidemic scabies and acute glomerulohephritis in Trinidad. *Lancet*, **i**, 249
16. Allen, B. R. (1972). Scabies and acute glomerulonephritis. *Lancet*, **i**, 434
17. Paterson, W. D., Allen, B. R. and Berridge, G. W. (1973). Norwegian scabies during immunosuppression therapy. *Br. Med. J.*, **4**, 211
18. Espy, P. D. and Jolly, M. W. (1976). Norwegian scabies. *Arch. Dematol.*, **112**, 193
19. Ingram, J. T. (1951). Ward epidemic from Norwegian scabies. *Br. J. Dermatol.*, **63**, 311
20. Buchan, W. (1766). *Domestic Medicine.* (London)
21. Hellier, F. F. (1939). Environment and constitution in dermatology. *Trans. St. John's Hosp Derm. Soc. (Lon.)*, **28**, 52
22. Danby, P. R., Church, R. E. and Sneddon, I. B. (1967). Eradicating scabies (letter). *Br. Med. J.*, **1**, 496
23. Shrank, A. B. and Alexander, S. L. (1967). Scabies: another epidemic? *Br. Med. J.*, **1**, 669
24. Haydon, J. R. and Caplan, R. M. (1971). Epidemic scabies. *Arch. Dermatol.*, **103**, 168
25. Schirren, J. M. (1970). Die Scabies, Eine Epidemiologische Studie. *Der Hautarzt*, **21**, 170
26. Epstein, E. (1966). Scabies, ten years later. *Arch Dermatol.*, **93**, 60
27. Hellier, F. F. (1966). Incidence of scabies (letter). *Arch. Dermatol.*, **93**, 634
28. MacMillen, A. L. (1972). Unusual features of scabies associated with topical fluorinated steroids. *Br. J. Dermatol*, **87**, 496
29. Schenone, H., Falaha, F., Szekely, R. *et al.* (1971). La sarna en pediatria. *Revista Chileanádi Pediatria*, **42**, 561

30. Nair, B. K. H., Joseph, A., Narayanan, P. I. and Chacko, K. V. (1973). Epidemiology of scabies. *Ind. J. Derm. Vener.*, **39**, 101
31. Church, R. E. and Knowelden, J. (1978). Scabies in Sheffield: A family infestation. *Br. Med. J.*, **1**, 761
32. Kanaaneh, H. A. K., Rabi, S. A. and Badarneh, S. M. (1976). Eradication of a large scabies outbreak using community-wide health education. *Amer. J. Public Health*, **66**, 564
33. Kutzer, E. and Grunberg, W. (1969). Zur Frage der Ubertrazung Tierischer Sarcoptesraaden auf den Menschen Berliner und Münchenen. *Tierarztliche Wochenschrift*, **52**, 311
34. Smith, E. B. and Claypole, T. F. (1967). Canine scabies in dogs and humans. *J. Amer. Med. Assoc.*, **199**, 59
35. Thomsett, L. R. (1968). Mite infestations of man contracted from dogs and cats. *Br. Med. J.*, **2**, 93
36. Davies, J. H. T. (1941). Cat itch. *Br. J. Dermatol.*, **53**, 18
37. Humphreys, N. (1958). *Cheyletiella parasitovax* infestation of the dog. *Vet. Rec.*, **70**, 442
38. Foxx, T. S. and Ewing, S. A. (1969). Morphological features, behaviour and life history of *Cheyletiella yasguri*. *Am. J. Vet. Res.*, **30**, 269
39. Hewitt, M., Walton, G. S. and Waterhouse, M. (1971). Pet animal infestations and human skin lesions. *Br. J. Dermatol.*, **85**, 215
40. De Oreo, G. A. (1958). Pigeons acting as vector in acariasis caused by *Dermanyssus gallinae*. *Arch. Dermatol.*, **77**, 422
41. Sulzberger, M. B. and Kaminstein, I. (1936). Avian itch mites as a cause of human dermatoses. *Arch. Dermatol. Syph.*, **33**, 60
42. Charlesworth, E. N. and Clegern, R. W. (1977). Tropical rat mite dermatitis. *Arch. Dermatol.*, **113**, 937
43. Fairburn, E. A. and Frain Bell, W. (1956). *Bdellonyssus bacoti* as a causal agent of cutaneous disease. *Br. J. Dermatol.*, **68**, 350
44. Riechers, R. and Kopt, A. W. (1969). Cutaneous infestation with *Demodex follicularis* in man. *J. Invest. Dermatol.*, **52**, 103
45. Muller, G. H. and Kirk, R. W. (1976). *Small Animal Dermatology*. 2nd Ed. (Philadelphia: W. B. Saunders) p. 353
46. Ayres, S. Jr. (1930). *Pityriasis folliculorum (Demodex)*. *Arch. Dermatol. Syph.*, **21**, 19
47. Ayres, S. Jr. and Mihan, R. (1967). Rosacea-like demodicidosis involving the eyelids. *Arch. Dermatol.*, **95**, 63
48. Spickett, S. G. (1962). Aetiology of rosacea (letter). *Br. Med. J.*, **1**, 1625
49. Booth, B. H. and Jones, R. W. (1954). Mites in industry. *Arch. Dermatol Syph.*, **69**, 531
50. Bagnall, B. and Rook, A. (1977). Arthropods and the skin. In: Rook, A. (ed.), *Recent Advances in Dermatology No. 4*, pp. 59–90. (Edinburgh: Churchill Livingstone)
51. Barnham, M. (1977). Human tick infestation in Britain (letter). *Br. Med. J.*, **2**, 1288
52. Rook, A., Wilkinson, D. S. and Ebling, F. J. G. (1972). *Textbook of Dermatology*. 2nd ed. p. 868. (Oxford: Blackwell)
53. Goldman, L. (1963). Tick bite granuloma. Failure of prevention of lesion by excision of tick bite area. *Am. J. Trop. Med.*, **12**, 246
54. Marshall, J. (1967). Ticks and the human skin. *Dermatologica*, **135**, 60
55. Schmitt, N. Bowmer, E. J. and Gregson, J. D. (1969). Tick paralysis in British Columbia. *Can. Med. Ass. J.*, **100**, 417
56. Darrow, G. L. (1974). Tick bite paralysis in a six-year-old girl. *Postgrad. Med.*, **56**, 187
57. Hollstrom, E. (1958). Penicillin treatment of *erythema chronicum migrans afzelius*. *Acta Dermat-venereol.*, **38**, 285
58. Degos, R., Touraine, R. and Arouete, J. (1962). *Erythema chronicum migrans*: discussion of rickettsial origin. *Ann. Dermat. Syph.*, **89**, 247
59. Varma, M. G. R. (1962). Transmission of relapsing fever spirochaetes by ticks. In: D. R. Arthur (ed.) *Aspects of Disease Transmission by Ticks* (London: Zoological Soc.). pp. 61–82
60. Davison, G., Naubauer, C. and Hurst, E. W. (1948). Meningo-encephalitis in man due to Louping-ill virus. *Lancet*, **ii**, 453
61. Harasek, G. (1974). Zeckenenzephalitis in Kindesalter. *Dtsch. Med. Wschr.*, **99**, 1965

4
Head Lice

R. J. DONALDSON

INTRODUCTION

Head louse infestation occurs throughout the world but evidence suggests that it has a greater prevalence in the Western world. This may seem a paradox to those who believe that the problem disappears with improved standards of hygiene in a more affluent society. It is discouraging that valuable manpower resources, which could be better deployed, are engaged in searching out those who harbour this unwanted parasite. Yet because of its high degree of specialization the louse is very vulnerable. The objectives of this chapter are to review the present state of knowledge and indicate ways in which man might rid himself once and for all of this persistent parasite.

CLASSIFICATION

There are two Orders of lice: the biting lice (Mallophaga) and the sucking lice (Anoplura). Most authorities agree that they both belong to the Order Phthiraptera.

The Mallophaga are the most primitive of lice; feeding on skin and feather debris, they probably had their origins as parasites of birds. From these biting lice, the sucking Order evolved, by adapting their biting mouths to piercing and sucking stylets so that they became dependent for nourishment solely on blood.

The Anoplura are parasites exclusively of mammals and two genera of lice infest man, *Phthirus* and *Pediculus*, although only one species of each is involved. When man began to wear clothes and his hair became restricted to the head, axillary and pubic areas, human lice underwent further refinements. The crab louse (*Phthirus pubis*) adapted to live on the hairy parts around the human genitalia, whilst the body louse migrated to clothing, returning to its host for food. The head louse became essentially a scalp-dweller and specialized to such a degree that its survival depends on it being in almost continual contact with its source of food and warmth.

In 1778 De Greer described two varieties of *Pediculus humanus* as *Pediculus humanus corporis* (the body louse) and *Pediculus humanus capitis* (the head louse). (The International Zoological code name for the body louse is now *Pediculus humanus humanus*.)

There has been considerable argument about whether the head louse and the body louse are separate species, subspecies or varieties of a single species. This area has been investigated by Busvine[1], who obtained body lice from naturally infested vagrants and head lice from infested schoolchildren and maintained colonies in captivity, using small gauze-bottomed pill boxes attached to the skin of his ankles. This contact was maintained only during the day for the body louse colonies, but continuously for the head lice, to prevent the high proportion of deaths which occurred when they were not in continuous contact with their source of food. Body lice were found to be, on average, larger in all dimensions, but there was overlap so that occasionally, for example, a large head louse exceeded the size of a small body louse. Thus it was possible to distinguish populations of the two forms, but it was not possible to identify every individual with certainty. The colonies were maintained by Busvine for two years (45 generations) and kept their distinctiveness. Kelin and Nuttall[2] had previously claimed that head lice, after being carried on the body for a few generations, lost their head lice characteristics and became typical body lice. The stringent segregation maintained by Busvine in his experiments now clearly seems to have dispelled this earlier theory.

A further feature of specialization in the louse relates to modification of the legs to grasp hairs of different cross-sectional shape. It has been observed that lice infesting the hair of negroes, which is oval in cross-section, find difficulty in transferring to the cylindrical cross-section of the hair of the Caucasian. Inferences have been made that there are subspecies of lice which have developed to infest different races and a nomenclature has been devised to deal with this. For example, *Pediculus humanus nigritorum* denotes the head louse infesting negroes.

However, the alternative view holds that such forms are not genetically distinct and that all intermediate shades can be found. The widespread migration of man would tend to militate against the establishment of geographical races of lice.

HISTORY

There is strong evidence that the head louse evolved along with man. Evidence of such a coexistence dates back many centuries. The eggs (nits) of head lice have been found on the hair of an Egyptian mummy. In the New World, lice have also occurred since ancient times. Nits have been found on pre-Columbian Peruvian mummies and on the hairs of prehistoric American

Indian mummies from the southwestern United States that are up to 4000 years old[3].

There are numerous references to the louse in literature from the time of the Greek classics. The famous English diarist, Samuel Pepys, is often quoted for his entries in the 1660s when he was 'vexed cruelly' by his Westminster barber for supplying him with a periwig infested with nits.

About a century later Scotland's immortal bard, Robert Burns, penned a poem whilst he watched a louse move across a lady's bonnet during a sermon in the kirk:

> 'Ye ugle, creepin, blastit wonner,
> Detested, shunned by saunt an' sinner,
> How daur ye set your fit upon her,
> Sae fine a lady.
> Gae somewhere else and seek your dinner
> On some poor body.'

BIOLOGY

In order to deal with the problems of control of head infestation it is essential to understand basic biological facts about the head louse.

Pediculus humanus capitis is a highly specialized host-specific parasite. For all practical purposes it is found only on the hair of the head of human beings.

The head louse (Figure 4.1) is about the size of the head of a matchstick (2–4 mm long). The male is slightly smaller than the female and has larger front legs with a thicker claw which is used to hold the hind legs of the female during copulation. Unlike the body louse, it is not equipped to live in clothing nor is it found on household pets like cats and dogs. The louse lives close to the scalp for warmth, moisture and food, and in the case of females, a place to lay eggs. It can move quickly and is difficult to see because of its greyish colour and tendency to blend with the shading of the hair of the host. Its three pairs of legs are especially modified to grasp the hair in a highly successful claw-like fashion. The louse has poor eyesight but a highly developed sense of touch. The two antennae are the sense organs and wave characteristically as the louse moves. Copulation takes place with the male beneath the female and they remain coupled for some time afterward and can feed in this position. The normal lifespan is about 30 days but few survive in the natural state for so long. The fertilized female lays about 6–8 eggs every 24 hours, mostly at night when the head of the host is still.

The female louse prepares a hair shaft very close to the scalp by squeezing on to it a glue-like substance similar in composition to hair itself. She then lays the egg which becomes firmly attached to the hair. Only one egg is laid on a hair shaft and, unlike its cousin the body louse, the head louse does not lay eggs on clothing. The egg is oval in shape and has a translucent pearly white

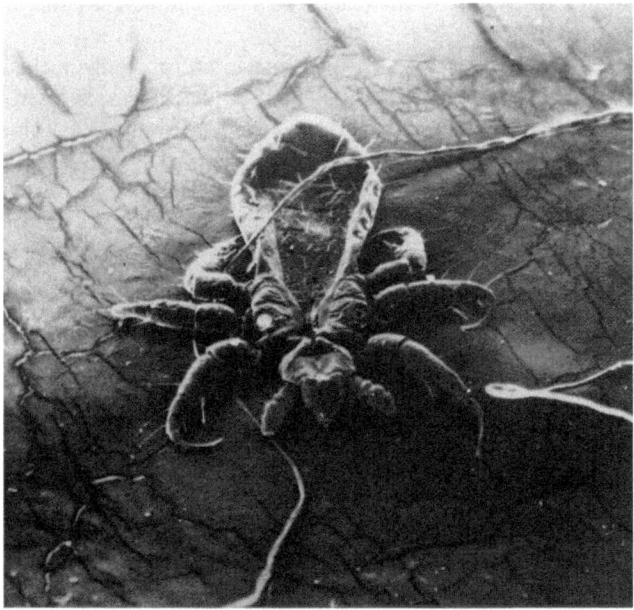

Figure 4.1 *Pediculus humanus capitis*, head louse, ×35

appearance. It measures about 0.8 mm by 0.3 mm and is easily seen with the naked eye. Temperature and moisture levels are critical in hatching the eggs. Few louse eggs will hatch at a temperature of under 22 °C and at that temperature probably less than 10% of eggs hatch in under 15 days. However, almost 90% would be expected to hatch within 7 days if at 34 °C. Careful inspection shows the developing embryo within the egg. The upper end of the egg has a flat lid with cavities which allows the embryo access to air. When the young louse in the egg has sufficiently developed it pushes its mouthparts through the membrane which encloses it into the air space in the egg cap. Air is then swallowed and passes through the louse and collects at its rear end. The young louse (nymph) is thus propelled from the egg shell by compressed air. The shell remains empty and fixed to the hair. Any nits found on hair more than a few centimetres from the scalp must, therefore, be either empty shells that have hatched or dead embryos.

Almost immediately after hatching, the nymph has its first meal of blood. The nymph is similar in appearance to the adult except in its size, but it must go through three stages of development, each separated by a moult before becoming an adult 10 or 11 days after hatching. Two days after reaching maturity the female is ready to lay eggs. The head louse feeds only on human blood. The feeding operation is carried out by the modified mouthparts of the louse which have their resting position within a pouch in the head. A series of curved teeth around the mouth fasten onto the skin, three small stylets pierce the skin of the host, and saliva passes into the wound through a central tube in the proboscis. This prevents the blood from clotting and is probably the cause of the irritation of the host's skin which classically occurs some hours later. The louse has a poorly developed defence mechanism and is easily killed by mechanical trauma, thus the comb is its worst enemy. It is also very sensitive to variations in the temperature of the host. Lice are known to leave the head of an individual with high pyrexia and at the time of death.

Perhaps the intimate association of the head louse is best illustrated by Maunder's analogy[4] that compares the outer hair of the human head to the outer atmosphere of the earth—barren, arid, cold and hostile.

MODE OF TRANSMISSION OF INFESTATION

The mode of transfer is almost certainly by the louse walking from one host's head to another. Under normal circumstances lice do not leave the host's scalp which is their source of food and warmth, so that the assumption is that lice will move to another host only when the hosts' heads are very close together. Schools provide the opportunity for the spread of infestation from one child to another during the close personal contact which occurs in the classroom and at play. Lice which fall off human heads can be disregarded as a source of spread because they are usually weak, old, or injured. There is little evidence to show that lice are transferred by headgear or combs. Similarly, other wearing apparel, furniture, seats in trains or theatres are unimportant as a source of infestation. Stray hairs bearing nits would seem to be an unusual method in view of what has been said about the hatching process.

In spite of this lack of evidence some North American authorities still continue to advise the sterilization of all personal clothing, bedclothes and bedding of the infested person and the disinfection of combs, hairbrushes, etc. They also recommend that undergarments and nightwear should be changed daily. Cleaning of toilet seats and vacuuming upholstered furniture, rugs and floors, laudable though these measures may be, are totally irrelevant when preventing transmission of head lice.

PREVALENCE

Great Britain

Data on the prevalence of head infestation on a national scale are scanty and are mainly available from British sources. The evacuation of children in England from the large cities to rural areas at the outbreak of World War II (in 1939) revealed a highly unsatisfactory state of lousiness amongst the evacuees. This had not been revealed by official data and caused considerable concern.

Mellanby[5] carried out a study in 1940 to clarify the problem. His data were derived from records of some 60 000 patients in 32 hospitals, mostly those which treated patients with infectious diseases. These hospitals were situated in large cities, smaller towns and rural areas. He believed that if hospitals, particularly in cities, treated some wealthy patients then the sample would be reasonably representative of the whole population.

The main conclusions from the survey were as follows (Figures 4.2 and 4.3):

   (i) a very high degree of infestation existed in industrial cities,
  (ii) girls were more frequently infested than boys,
 (iii) the highest rate of infestation was found amongst pre-school children,
 (iv) that infestation among boys decreased steadily from about three years of age (where over 40% were verminous) to young adulthood where levels were very low. In girls there was no such decrease before the age of 13 years and even after that age, there was still a considerable degree of lousiness,
  (v) little support was given to the idea that the aged are frequently verminous. Those over 70 years showed a percentage of lousiness similar to that of other adults,
 (vi) infestation rates in females aged 9–13 years reached a maximum of 62% in the most heavily infested city, while the lowest was 36%. In five out of the ten industrial cities, 50% of girls were found to be verminous,
(vii) the overall rate of infestation was 30.3%.

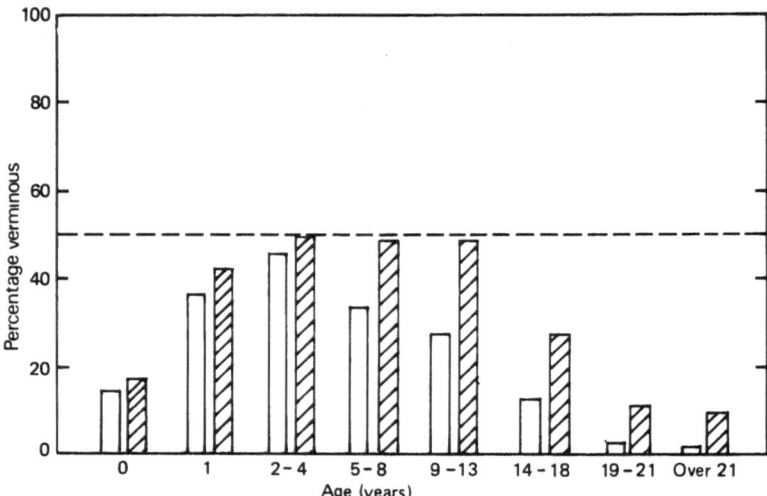

Figure 4.2 Percentage of individuals in ten industrial cities. White, males; Striped, females. 52,445 results. (Source: Mellanby[5])

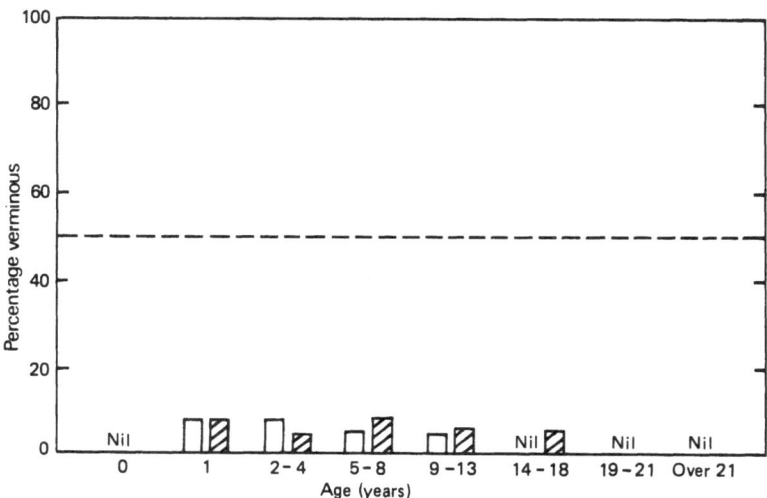

Figure 4.3 Percentage of individuals verminous in four southern rural countries. White, males; Striped, females. 2,522 results. (Source: Mellanby[5])

Mellanby's study provided an important basis for comparison despite the limitation that it depended on hospital records as a source of information and the fact that the sample could not have been representative of the population as a whole.

Smaller local surveys showed improvements after World War II in Britain but in the 1960s and early 1970s there was again concern about an apparent increase in prevalence. In 1969 Wilson[6] reported that in Glasgow infestation of girls entering school was as common as in the 1930s (10% had nits) and amongst boy entrants the prevalence had increased over the period from 1 to 4%. Routine statistics for England and Wales collected by the Department of Education and Science indicated during this period that there was a rising proportion of infested schoolchildren (see Table 4.1).

Unfortunately from these data it is not clear which children have been examined. Some have certainly been examined more than once. For example 10.6 million examinations were carried out in 1970 when the school population was 7.7 million.

A prospective survey of prevalence of head infestation was carried out in Teesside County Borough in north-east England in 1970 when statistics collected by school nurses indicated an infestation rate of 5.7% amongst schoolchildren. The study mainly considered schoolchildren between 5 and 11 years and the sample was stratified in three social areas—poor, intermediate and good. A sample of 3600 children was drawn at random from each stratum involving 40 schools. The overall rate of infestation was 15.7% and varied from

Table 4.1 The health of the schoolchild

Year	Number examined	Number lousy	Number of pupils on school register	% Rate of infestation
1938	14 586 091	444 967	5 035 276	3.05
1944	15 398 668	502 348	4 519 498	3.26
1945	13 560 068	482 188	5 022 068	3.55
1950	15 645 840	400 406	5 651 155	2.55
1951	15 357 865	347 544	5 737 698	2.26
1960	13 168 352	207 883	7 014 809	1.57
1961	12 500 954	200 655	7 042 873	1.60
1969	10 718 418	203 757	8 080 731	1.90
1970	11 323 111	237 818	8 284 923	2.10
1973	12 833 301	255 755	9 118 678	1.99
1974	11 028 442	223 824		2.02

Source: *Health of the Schoolchild*, 1939–45, 1950–51, 1960–61, 1969–70, 1973–74. HMSO, London. Compiled by Diane Oxley, BA.

23.3% in the poor area to 0.6% in the good area (Table 4.2). The study underlines the unreliability of routine data for deriving infestation rates and highlights head infestation as a correlate of disadvantage[7].

A national prevalence survey carried out in England in 1975 showed that head infestation was widespread amongst schoolchildren of all ages[8]. The sample was drawn from children attending primary and secondary schools in different geographical localities and the sampling method ensured that children from both urban and rural areas were represented. Primary schoolchildren (aged 5–11 years) were further classified in good, middle and poor zones according to the social background of the areas the schools served. This zoning was not performed for the secondary schoolchildren (aged 11–18 years), as many of their catchment areas were too large and heterogeneous.

Table 4.2 Percentage of primary schoolchildren with head infestation by social area, September 1970

Area	% Lice	% Nits	% Infested
Downtown	4.0	19.3	23.3
Intermediate	1.1	12.4	13.5
Suburban	0.3	0.3	0.6

Source: Donaldson[7]

Classes were chosen from each school as being representative in terms of age structures. Every child in the chosen class was examined by a member of a team of school nurses, all of whom had been given special instruction in the method to be used and had been told of the importance of recording every case of infestation, no matter how lightly the head was infested.

The survey had the great merit of simplicity as schoolchildren in England are normally frequently inspected by school nurses and, since data were collected about the child's form, it was easy to obtain age-bands of children, and information on social background was derived from the social zone of the school. The report, giving details of the method and analysis of the results, is obtainable from the Health Education Council, New Oxford Street, London, W.C.1. The results of the survey may be summarized as follows:

(1) The estimated overall prevalence of infestation was 2.45% (primary schools: 2.43%, secondary schools: 2.46%). The estimated total number of children infested was 193 806,

(2) Infestation was widespread amongst schoolchildren of all ages, but more so in the north than in the south, in urban more than in rural areas, the highest rate of all being observed amongst schoolchildren in the deprived central zones of the big cities (Figure 4.4).

(3) Girls were more frequently infested than boys (Figure 4.5),

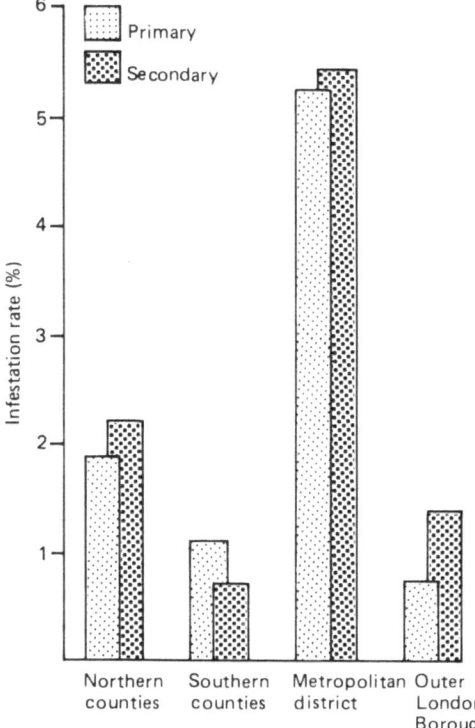

Figure 4.4 Infestation by type and authority. (Source: Donaldson[8])

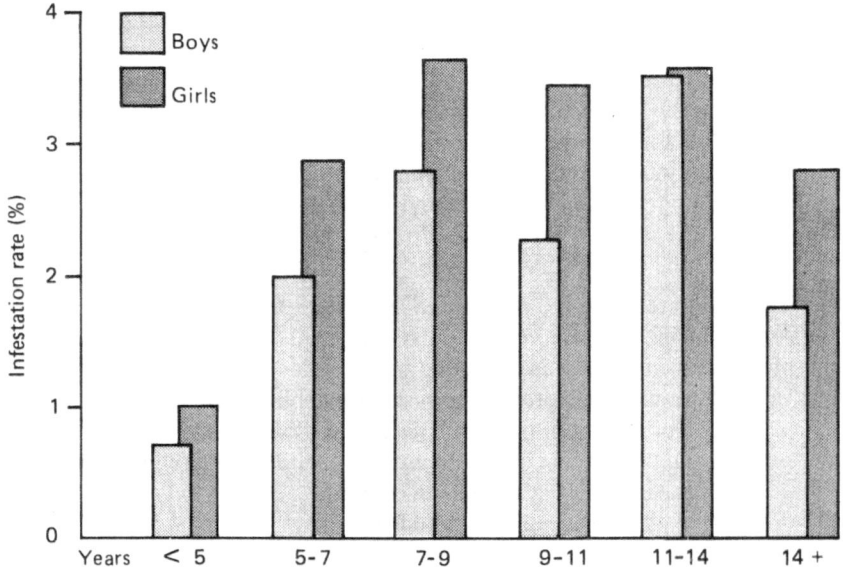

Figure 4.5　Infestation rate by age and sex. (Source: Donaldson[8])

(4) For both sexes the lowest rate of infestation was amongst children under five years and the highest amongst young teenagers.

The Americas

Differing prevalence of head infestation is well reviewed by Gratz[9]. He observed that very high rates of head lice infestation are reported in Canada and the USA. Surveys carried out by the US Center for Disease Control in three cities in the US revealed levels of infestation that ranged from 3% to 20% of the children surveyed. White children were more commonly infested than black.

Orkin (1974)[10] projected that there would be about 3 million cases of pediculosis (all species) in the USA in 1974, 50% more than in 1973.

At a symposium on head lice transmission and treatment held in 1976, there was speculation that there might be 6 million infestations with head lice in the USA at that time (Anon., 1976); this estimate was based on numbers of sales of pediculicides.

A large-scale survey was carried out in Chile in 1971 in which 53 556 persons were examined for the presence of head lice[11]. Most of those examined were schoolchildren. The general prevalence of infestation was 20% (17.3% for males and 22.5% for females). In general, levels of infestation were higher in groups of older people and amongst women rather than men. In persons over

20 years of age, there were twice as many women as men infested (women 14.7%; men 7.1%).

Europe (excluding Britain) and the Middle East

Bloomers (1978) (personal communication) reported circumstantial evidence which indicated an increase in prevalence of head louse infestation in Holland over recent years. The sales of commercial lotions had increased by 125% between 1971 and 1974. Moreover, 10 000 cases of infested children were reported to the Ministry of Health in 1974 but 14 000 in 1975. However, he pointed out that these records were far from complete and was therefore unable to quote a reliable national figure. He hinted that the increased prevalence might be due to resistance to gamma-benzene hexachloride and pointed out that, although lindane was used for 25 years, resistance to it was found only in 1977.

Gratz[12] reports that Lidror and Lifshitz[13] inspected several thousand children in schools in several villages in Israel and calculated a level of infestation of 39.5% in settlements of new immigrants from Eastern and North African countries. Infestation levels in schools in districts where the children were either those of old settlers or of immigrants from Western countries were only 3.3%.

Gratz also reported that in Libya 3000 cases of head lice infestation were seen in the Central Hospital of Tripoli during 1975 and that 19 000 patients attended the hospital for complications of head lice infestation, such as impetigo, out of a total of 203 932 outpatients[12]. It was estimated that 10% of the outpatients and 2% of the children attending a school health centre were infested and that the probable rate of head lice infestation for the entire country was 10 to 15 per hundred population.

One is left with the intriguing question as to why head infestation should be increasing. Perhaps it is too easy to attribute it solely to insect resistance and we should look instead to our heritage of infectious diseases surveillance which has demonstrated often enough that control of pests and diseases can only be achieved by constant vigilance.

SIGNS AND SYMPTOMS

Most infestations seen today tend to be light and in such cases symptoms are pruritus of the scalp and disturbance of sleep. With heavier infestation the effects of hundreds of bites by head lice, apart from causing local skin irritation, may give rise to mild pyrexia and muscular aches typically in the calves of the legs. With scratching it is common to get secondary infection which may produce cervical gland enlargement. Secondary infection may also arise from lice which carry impetigo-causing bacteria in their intestines and whose faeces may infect the wounds caused by scratching.

The commonly-described plaque, formed of pus and other debris on which fungal growth has occurred, is today seldom seen.

DIAGNOSIS

If someone, particularly a child or young person, presents an itchy scalp, impetigo, excoriation of the scalp or nape of the neck, it is important to suspect head infestation. The main diagnostic feature is the presence of eggs (nits) which are more frequently located behind the ears, although they may be found anywhere on the hair of the head. Eggs are unlikely to be 'live' if found on the hair more than a few centimetres from the scalp. They can be easily distinguished from seborrhoeic eczema (dandruff) because they are firmly attached to the shaft of the hair and, unlike dandruff, cannot be easily dislodged. Live lice are difficult to see. Diagnosis can be confirmed with the lens of a low-powered microscope. Misdiagnosis can occur where small pieces of scalp become glued to the hair, perhaps by hairspray[14].

EDUCATION PROGRAMME

It is important when dealing with the problem of infestation in the community to have an accurate method of measuring and monitoring levels of infestation. The method suggested in this chapter is accurate, simple and ideal for evaluating control measures.

The essential prerequisite for prevention and control is a well-planned public education campaign initially to dispel myths and misconceptions which surround the subject. This is no less true now than it was in 1941, when Mellanby[5] recommended that 'education of the public is the only method likely to produce permanent success'. In parts of England, mothers still believe that their children breed lice, almost echoing the medieval belief that 'lice are generated from the very flesh of men'. Even amongst professionals there is appalling ignorance. At a recent meeting with health workers in North America, I was astonished to learn that they believed that human head lice lived on cats and dogs.

Thus, it is to the professionals that the first stage of any education campaign should be directed. Experience has shown that physicians, nurses, pharmacists, teachers, health educators, and environmental health workers have much to learn.

Next must come the education of the general public in a simple and direct way, using posters, leaflets, lectures and visual aids. (Details of two suitable films are included at the end of the chapter). Our experience in Teesside showed that the use of anti-louse propaganda in the form of a letter and a leaflet to the parent of every schoolchild cut the level of infestation by half (see Figure 4.6). Public education is, indeed, a most effective insecticide.

Probably the greatest obstacle to the launching of a public education programme is the reluctance to discuss the subject openly. The unsavoury

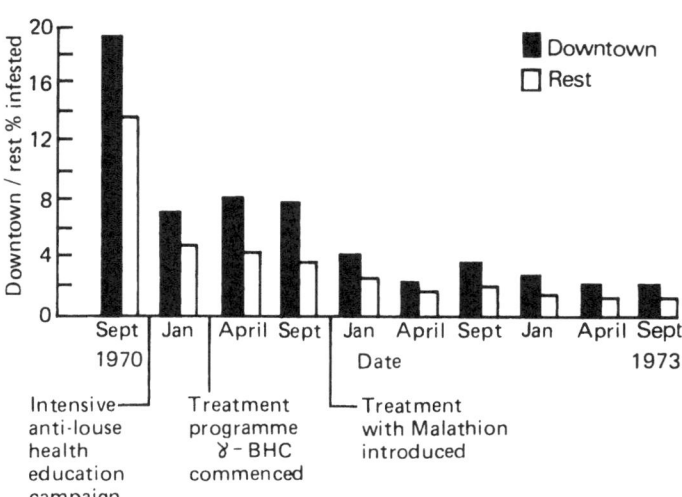

Figure 4.6 Head infestation levels amongst primary schoolchildren in deprived (downtown) areas and the rest of Teesside, September 1970–September 1973

nature of the topic has led to concealment of the problem by nations, communities, schools, families and individuals. There is a fear that if information were revealed, the image of a community or an individual would be tarnished.

INSECTICIDES

During their long association with man, many remedies have been advocated for head lice. However, during and after World War II, a considerable measure of success was achieved with the introduction of dichloro-diphenyl-trichloroethane (DDT) and gamma-benzene hexachloride (γ-BHC). Resistance to these insecticides has been reported since the late 1960s, particularly in the United Kingdom. This has almost certainly been a contributory factor to increased prevalence.

The resistance of head lice to insecticides is an hereditary characteristic and is due to contact with sublethal doses by their ancestors. Generally, resistant strains are selected into predominance by extensive prior use of insecticide. The wide range of insecticides in common use fall into just five groups, so that if an insect becomes resistant to one particular insecticide, it simultaneously acquires resistance to all other members of that group. The five are dichloro-diphenyl-trichloroethane (DDT), chlorodine— which includes gamma benzene hexachloride (γ-BHC)—organophosphorus, the carbamate groups and the pyrethroids.

When resistance is so strongly developed that control is seriously threatened, the only option is to change to an insecticide from a different group.

DDT has been employed in many countries as a general measure of louse control and, as a result, strains of lice resistant to DDT have emerged. Gamma-BHC has also been widely used for head infestation and resistance to it has also arisen. Maunder[15] reports resistance from over 20 different areas of Britain where γ-BHC or DDT were used against head lice. Concentrations of organochlorine insecticides tolerated by head lice from London proved to be well in excess of the dose found to be lethal to lice 20 years ago[16]. In clinical trials carried out in 1971, malathion was markedly superior in both initial cure and residual action to γ-BHC. Maunder[15] carried out his trials in three areas that were assessed to have low, intermediate and high chances of reinfestation. Details of the results are given in Table 4.3. He also demonstrated the lethal

Table 4.3 Comparison of residual effects of malathion and γ-BHC

Area	Reinfestation chances	Insecticide	Number treated	% with lice at 1–3 days	Number reinspected at 1 month	% with lice at 1 month (excluding those lousy at 1–3 days)
Exton	Low	0.5% malathion lotion	777	Nil	710	1.4
Stockton	Low	0.2% γ-BHC (Lorexane)	729	4.2	680	7.2
Middlesbrough	Intermediate	0.5% malathion lotion (Prioderm)	230	Nil	224	7.6
Middlesbrough	Intermediate	0.2% γ-BHC	247	10.1	236	28.1
Stepney	High	0.5% malathion lotion (Prioderm)	113	Nil	86	4.6
Stepney	High	0.2% γ-BHC lotion	71	10.0	60	41.7

Source: modified from Maunder[15]

effect to lice of hair clippings from children treated with malathion between 1 and 6 weeks previously. Neither DDT nor γ-BHC are ovicidal; the eggs still hatch so that a further treatment may be required 8 or 10 days later. Another disadvantage of the older treatments is that neither DDT nor γ-BHC have any significant lasting effect when used as shampoos and perform little better as lotions, so that a person will have no residual protection after treatment if he comes into contact with further infestation. Both malathion and carbaryl have proved very effective in treating head infestation. There is as yet no firm evidence of resistance to these two insecticides, and moreover they are ovicidal and bond onto the hair to give a residual effect. This appears to provide substantial protection for up to 6 weeks after the initial application.

One drawback of malathion is that even slight hydrolysis results in the release of foul-smelling mercaptans. Fortunately, this problem has been overcome with the proprietary preparations which have been formulated into lotions. These newer insecticides act on the nerve junctions of the louse and cause paralysis. Death is rapid, particularly with carbaryl.

The lethal effect of the insecticide depends on two factors, the concentration of the insecticide and the time of contact. Maunder[4] argues convincingly that this is a basis for choosing lotion in preference to shampoo for treatment. He concludes that a lotion containing 0.5% insecticide can give an effective dose to the insect one thousand times greater than that of a shampoo containing 1% when equal quantities are applied. He also stresses the importance of overkill to avoid the emergence of a resistant louse population, pointing out that the effects of an insecticide in a population of insects bear a logarithmic relationship to the dose employed. The moderate dose required to kill 90% of the louse population must be multiplied many times to produce a 100% kill.

However, a small but well-designed trial carried out in East London comparing the results of treatment of infested schoolchildren with either an alcoholic lotion containing 0.5% malathion or a cream shampoo containing 1% malathion found them to be equally effective. Although children were randomly allocated to one or other treatment group, the lotion group were treated by trained staff at a centre, whereas the shampoo group were dealt with by giving their parents shampoo with which to treat the children at home. Twenty-eight children were treated with shampoo and 22 with lotion. The children were inspected again between 7 and 14 days and after 6 weeks. There was a virtual 100% cure rate in both groups and none of the patients was infested when examined 6 weeks after a single treatment. One patient treated with shampoo had live eggs when inspected after 7 days and was given a further supply of shampoo for home treatment. The child was cured when inspected a week later. This was presumably due to initial non-treatment or inadequate treatment. The results are shown in Table 4.4.[17].

Table 4.4 Comparative trial of shampoo and lotion

	Treatment	
	Prioderm cream shampoo	Prioderm lotion
Number of patients	28	22
Number free of infestation at one/two weeks	27	22
Number free of infestation at six weeks	28	22

Source: Preston and Fry[17]

TOXICITY OF INSECTICIDES

The toxicity of the various insecticides used in the treatment of head infestation is frequently raised in discussion with health workers. Most of the information given here has been obtained from World Health Organisation sources[18, 19-21]. The four insecticides (DDT, γ-BHC, malathion and carbaryl) referred to are discussed and the BHC isomer considered is lindane which is still widely used in treatment.

DDT

Structural formula

Biochemical aspects

DDT is only slightly absorbed by the skin. If taken orally some absorption may occur and a certain amount accumulates in the fat particularly in females. DDT is also secreted in milk. Its toxic effects involve the central nervous system and cause death in animals usually as a result of respiratory arrest. The effects of DDT have been studied extensively in several species of animals, in all of which it has had an effect on the liver; the rat is particularly susceptible. In man oral doses equivalent to 0.5 mg/kg body weight daily for as long as eighteen months appear to result in no harmful effects. Nevertheless DDT accumulates in the fat and the eventual consequence of it being mobilized should be considered. However, only the slight degree of absorption which occurs through the skin is of relevance in the treatment of head infestation, although children are particularly susceptible.

Lindane

Structural formula

Biochemical aspects

Lindane is absorbed from the digestive tract and also by the skin. Once absorbed, lindane is distributed to various tissues and organs accumulating above all in fat depots, liver and kidneys. The unchanged compound is found in milk. Growing animals are particularly susceptible to its toxicity. Lindane, from the point of view of acute toxicity, is the most toxic of all isomers present in the technical hexachlorocyclohexanes. It is a neurotropic poison affecting

Table 4.5 Acute oral and dermal toxicity of insecticides to adult rats

Compound	Oral LD_{50} (mg/kg)		Dermal LD_{50} (mg/kg)	
	Male rats	Female rats	Male rats	Female rats
DDT	113	118	—	2510
Lindane	88	91	1000	900
Malathion	1375	1000	> 4444	> 4444
Carbaryl	850	500	4000	4000

Source: Selected data from Gaines[22]

the central nervous system, causing first excitement and later depression, particularly of the respiratory centre.

It has been studied in a variety of animal species and has proved to be a cumulative poison causing hepatic and renal lesions as well as disturbances of the central nervous system. As will be seen from Table 4.5, from the viewpoint of acute toxicity it is the most toxic of the four compounds considered both by the oral and dermal routes.

Malathion

Structural formula

$$CH_3O \diagdown P \diagup \diagdown \; SCH.COOC_2H_5$$

$$CH_3O \diagup \quad \quad \quad \; | $$

$$CH_2COOC_2H_5$$

(P double-bonded to S; two CH_3O groups on phosphorus; $SCH.COOC_2H_5$ with $CH_2COOC_2H_5$ below)

Biochemical aspects

Malathion may be absorbed by inhalation, from the gastrointestinal tract or through the intact skin. It acts indirectly as a cholinesterase inhibitor after metabolism to malaoxon, the oxygen analogue. It is only very slightly secreted in milk. It is not accumulated in body tissues. No increased incidence of cancer has been reported in several long-term dietary studies in rats. In man most cases of poisoning have been associated with gross misuse, usually involving accidental or suicidal ingestion of the compound, or have occurred in the occupational situation when safety precautions have not been observed.

Carbaryl

Structural formula

Biochemical aspects

Absorbed by all routes although absorption by the skin is slow as shown by low dermal toxicity, it acts as an inhibitor of cholinesterase which is relatively rapidly reversible, the half-life of the inhibited enzyme being about 30 minutes. It does not accumulate in mammalian tissues. Excretion is largely in the urine. Long-term dietary studies of rats and mice show no increase in tumour incidence.

General observations on toxicity

In reading through the large number of sudies on acute and chronic toxicity of these four compounds it was encouraging to find that the two newer insecticides which I recommend for the treatment of head infestation are less toxic than those they replace.

TREATMENT OF PATIENTS

From the evidence now available the insecticides of choice for treatment of head infestation are malathion and carbaryl. Gamma-BHC and DDT should be regarded as obsolete. Lotions are the treatment of choice, but shampoo is often more acceptable to patients and provides a satisfactory alternative.

Whichever regime of treatment is used, it cannot be too strongly stressed that the treatment must be carried out confidentially, particularly with children, to avoid causing psychological trauma to the child. Both treatments with lotion and shampoo are easy to administer.

When treating with lotion, the hair should not be washed since greasy hair appears to enhance the bonding process of the insecticides, thus accentuating the residual effect. The lotion is sprinkled onto the hair and rubbed gently into the scalp, care being taken to avoid getting the lotion into the eyes. It is important to ensure that both hair and scalp are thoroughly moistened, especially around the ears and the nape of the neck. The hair should dry naturally and no heat should be used, not even a hairdrier. This is not so much because of the inflammability of the spirit-based lotion, but to prevent the insecticide being degraded by heat. The hair may be washed 12 to 24 hours later.

In the case of shampoo treatment, the application is similar to that of an ordinary shampoo. The hair is wetted thoroughly with warm water, the shampoo is applied and rubbed into all parts of the scalp. It should then be left for 4 to 5 minutes, after which the hair is rinsed thoroughly with clean water and the procedure repeated.

Fine toothcombing with a metal comb is frequently carried out to remove the nits, but it is a painful process and may be made easier when the hair is wet. However, this is purely a cosmetic exercise because of the ovicidal effect of the insecticide. A single treatment usually suffices. The insecticide may be used if impetigo is present and is not contraindicated in the presence of eczema or psoriasis. The treatment of head infestation must always precede antibiotic therapy.

The reservoir of infestation is frequently the family, so when an infested child is detected at school it is important that the *whole* family should be treated. It is here that the shampoo could prove useful because a higher degree of compliance can be expected in adults.

The ovicidal effect of the insecticide sometimes produces changes in the appearance of the eggs that are left attached to the hair. The colour may change because of maceration of the embryo (the 'red nit') or the shell may collapse (the 'small nit').

CONCLUSION

There are those who argue that head infestation should be dismissed as a trivial health problem in the context of the more serious conditions of today. It is hoped that this attitude will not prevail. We now have a splendid opportunity to rid ourselves once and for all of this unwanted parasite. Very effective treatment is now available. If the parasite survives long enough to acquire resistance, this will be because of a conspiracy of silence. The unsavoury nature of the subject has led to concealment not only by individuals and families but by schools and whole communities. What is urgently needed is a well-informed education campaign to dispel the myths and misconceptions surrounding this subject. In this we all have a part to play.

References

1. Busvine, J. R. (1976). *Insects, Hygiene and History*, pp. 42–44. (Athlone Press)
2. Kelin, D. and Nuttall, G. H. F. (1919). Relations of head and body lice of man. *Parasitology,* **11,** 279
3. Cloudsley-Thompson, J. L. (1976). *Insects and History*, p. 104. (Weidenfeld and Nicholson)
4. Maunder, J. W. (1977). Human lice—biology and control. *Roy. Soc. Health J.,* **97,** 29

5. Mellanby, K. (1941). The incidence of head lice in England. *Med. Officer*, **65**, 39
6. Wilson, T. S. (1969). *Med. Officer*, **122**, 125
7. Donaldson, R. J. (1974). *Head infestation—a community problem*, pp. 2–7. (Napp Laboratories)
8. Donaldson, R. J. (1975). *The Head Louse in England: Prevalence amongst Schoolchildren.* Health Education Council Report
9. Gratz, N. G. (1976). *The Epidemiology of Louse Infestations.* (Geneva: World Health Organization)
10. Orkin, M. (1974). *Pediculosis Today.* (Minn. Med., Oct. 1974)
11. Schenone, M., Falah, F., Villarroel, F., Rojas, A., Széksly, R., Rajo, M. and Palomino, H. (1973) La infestación por *Pediculus humanus capitis* en Santiago de Chili. *Bol. Chile Parasit.*, **28**, 31
12. Gratz, N. G. (1973). The current status of louse infestations throughout the world. In: *Proc. Int. Symp. Control of Lice and Louse-borne Diseases*, pp. 25–31, *PAHO Sci. Pub. no. 263*, Washington
13. Lidror, R. and Lifshitz, Y. (1965). A new method for lice control in Israel. *Public Health (Israel)*, **8**, 1
14. Editorial (1975). A nit or not a nit. *Br. Med. J.*, **1**, 354
15. Maunder, J. W. (1971). Use of malathion in the treatment of lousy children. *Comm. Med.*, **126**, 145
16. Maunder, J. W. (1971). Resistance to organochlorine insecticides in head lice and trials using alternative compounds. *Med. Officer*, **125**, 27
17. Preston, S. and Fry, L. (1977). A comparative trial of a malathion lotion and malathion shampoo in the treatment of head lice. *Roy. Soc. Health J.*, **97**, 6, 291
18. Evaluation of the toxicity of pesticide residues in food. *FAO Meeting Report* No. PL/1963/13 (mimeographed); *WHO/Food Add./23/1964* (mimeographed)
19. Evaluation of the toxicity of pesticide residues in food. *Report of the second joint meeting of the FAO Committee on Pesticides in Agriculture and the WHO Expert Committee on Pesticide Residues*, FAO Meeting Report No. PL/1965/10; WHO/Food Add./26.65
20. Data Sheets on Pesticides, No. 3, January 1975. *Carbaryl.* WHO/FAO VBC/DS/75.3
21. Data Sheets on Pesticides, No. 29. *Malathion.* WHO/FAO VBC/DS/77.29
22. Gaines, T. B. (1960). *Toxicol. Appl. Pharmacol.*, **2**, 88
23. Donaldson, R. J. (1975). *Equalities and Inequalities in Health*, p. 138. (London: Academic Press)

Recommended films

War to the Last Itch

16 mm. Colour. 17½ mins. (Made by C2M Film Productions, 1973.) Describes in detail the incidence, biology and prevention of head lice. Hire charge £4.50. Purchase price £125.00, plus VAT.

Available from: Peter Darvill Associates Ltd.,
　　　　　　　　280 Chartridge Lane,
　　　　　　　　Chesham, Bucks, HP5 2SG.
　　　　　　　　(Tel. 02405 3643)

On Your Own Head Be It

16 mm. Colour. 1977. An educational film on the methods by which a head lice campaign should be operated to ensure total eradication. (Currently available on hire—free of charge.)

Available from: Prioderm Information Service,
              Napp Laboratories Ltd.,
              Hill Farm Avenue,
              Watford, WD2 7RA.
              (Tel. Garston 75255)

5
Nematodes

R. MULLER

INTRODUCTION

The nematodes constitute a large group of unsegmented roundworms which occupy almost every habitat in all parts of the world. They must be regarded as one of the most successful groups in the animal kingdom, whether success is measured in numerical terms or by adaptability.

A remarkable feature of the group is that they show great uniformity of structure, whether they are microscopic free-living forms in soil or freshwater or parasitic worms of plants or animals which can be up to 60 cm in length. All nematodes also share the same basic life-cycle comprising an egg stage, four larval stages, and adult worms.

About a dozen nematode species are important parasites of man, while a further fifty may on occasion take up abode in the human body.

Some of these nematode infections are widespread and are found in a high proportion of the population of the world (*Ascaris* about 30%, *Trichuris* and hookworms 15%, filariae 7%). In general, they are pathogens only where standards of living and of hygiene are low. A few, such as *Enterobius* and *Trichinella*, are more common in the Western world than in developing countries and others, such as *Strongyloides* and *Ascaris*, may always be potentially dangerous, so it is important that the clinician and laboratory technologist can recognize and confirm nematode infections.

A typical nematode is cylindrical, tapering at both ends, and covered with an impermeable multilayered proteinaceous cuticle. There are few of the external protuberances which characterize the trematodes and cestodes, although there may be expansions of the cuticle at the head or tail end. Beneath the cuticle is a layer of muscle cells and lying between this layer and the gut is a fluid-filled body cavity with a high hydrostatic pressure.

The sexes are separate and the male is usually smaller than the female and is distinguished in its external appearance by the structure of the tail.

The nematodes have been divided into two groups; the first includes all those forms which are confined primarily to the gastrointestinal tract, and the second, those which are important pathologically as tissue parasites (*Trichinella* has been included among the tissue parasites, despite the fact that the adult is found in the intestine, because it is the larvae in the muscles that do most damage). It will be seen from Table 5.1 that most members of the former group have a direct life cycle while in the latter group an intermediate host is required.

In temperate climates the intestinal nematodes are very much more common than the tissue parasites. However, one group of tissue nematodes, the filariae, are widespread and important causes of morbidity in tropical countries.

CLASSIFICATION OF NEMATODES AFFECTING MAN

Phylum Nematoda

Elongate cylindrical parasites with separate sexes. Unsegmented with an intestine, mouth and anus. Have a fluid-filled body cavity (pseudocoelom).

Subclass Secernentea

Phasmids (paired, single-celled, glandular or sensory organelles at tail end, opening to exterior by pore) present.

Order Rhabditida
Parasites of ileum. Have alternation of parasitic and free-living generations. Parasitic females parthenogenetic. 'Rhabditoid' type oesophagus in free-living generation. Some forms pass larvae instead of eggs in faeces. *Strongyloides*.

Order Oxyurida
Parasites of colon or rectum. Oesophagus with characteristic bulb. Eggs flattened on one side. One spicule in male. *Enterobius*.

Order Ascaridida
Parasites of small intestine. Large stout nematodes. Thick-shelled eggs with unsegmented ovum passed in faeces. Oesophagus not divided into short muscular and long glandular portions. *Ascaris (Toxocara, Toxascaris, Anisakis*—larvae only in man).

Order Strongyloida
Parasites of intestine or respiratory system. Eggs with thin shell and containing segmenting ovum when passed. Male with caudal bursa; spicules of male tail similar. First stage larva has 'rhabditoid' oesophagus.

Superfamily Ancylostomatoidea
Buccal capsule subglobular. No lips. Parasites of small intestine. *Necator, Ancylostoma.*

Superfamily Trichostrongyloidea
Buccal capsule small or absent. Parasites of small intestine. *Trichostrongylus.*

Superfamily Metastrongyloidea
Caudal bursa often reduced. Parasites of respiratory system. (*Angiostrongylus*—larvae only in man).

Order Spirurida
Anterior end bilaterally symmetrical. Oesophagus divided into short anterior muscular and longer glandular portion. Parasites of stomach, oesophagus, or tissues and tissue spaces. Always transmitted by an invertebrate intermediate host ('vector').

Suborder Camallina

Superfamily Dracunculoidea
Female much larger than male. Parasites of connective tissues. First stage larva free-living; microcrustaceans as intermediate host. *Dracunculus.*

Suborder Spirurina

Superfamily Filarioidea
Parasites of tissues and tissue spaces. Transmitted by blood-feeding arthropod vectors; no free-living larval stage. Spicules dissimilar. All human parasites ovoviviparous with microfilaria larvae in blood or skin. *Wuchereria, Brugia, Loa, Dipetalonema, Mansonella, Onchocerca, Dirofilaria* (does not mature in man).

Subclass Adenophorea

Phasmids absent. Oesophagus non-muscular. Eggs usually have plug at either end or may be ovoviviparous. First stage larva infective to final host. *Trichuris, Trichinella.*

INTESTINAL NEMATODES

Strongyloides stercoralis

Geographical distribution

Strongyloidiasis occurs in most parts of the world in which the climate is warm and humid and is quite common both in southern Europe and in the southern

Table 5.1 Nematodes of medical importance

Mode of transmission	Species of nematode	Route of infection	Site of adult form	Geographical distribution
I. Intestinal parasites (No intermediate host)				
Contaminative	Enterobius vermicularis	Mouth	Large intestine	Cosmopolitan
Soil transmitted	Ascaris lumbricoides	Mouth	Small intestine	Cosmopolitan
	Trichuris trichiura	Mouth	Caecum	Cosmopolitan
	Ancylostoma duodenale	Skin or mouth	Small intestine	Tropics and subtropics
	Necator americanus	Skin	Small intestine	Tropics and subtropics
	Strongyloides stercoralis	Skin	Small intestine	Tropics and subtropics
	Trichostrongylus spp.	Mouth	Small intestine	Asia, Middle East, Africa
Abnormal or abortive infections	Ancylostoma spp. (Dermal larva migrans)	Skin		Asia, Africa, America, Pacific
	Toxocara (Visceral larva migrans)	Mouth	Liver, eye, brain, other organs (larva)	Cosmopolitan
II. Tissue parasites (intermediate host required)				
Meat transmitted	Trichinella spiralis	Mouth	Small intestine	Cosmopolitan
Fish transmitted	Anisakis	Mouth	Intestine wall (larva only in Man)	Europe, Japan, N. America
Snail transmitted	Angiostrongylus cantonensis	Snails and crustacea by mouth	Meninges (larva)	Pacific
Insect transmitted	Onchocerca volvulus	Simulium	Subcutaneous	Africa, Yemen, Central and South America
	Wuchereria bancrofti	Culex, Anopheles, and Aedes	Lymphatics	Asia, Africa, South America Pacific
	Brugia malayi	Mansonia	Lymphatics	South East Asia
	Loa loa	Chrysops	Subcutaneous	Africa (rain forest)
	Dipetalonema perstans	Culicoides	Peritoneal cavity	Africa, South America
	Dipetalonema streptocerca	Culicoides	Subcutaneous	Africa (rain forest)
	Mansonella ozzardi	Culicoides (?Simulium)	Peritoneal cavity	South America, West Indies

United States (10.7% prevalence in Rumania[1]; 4% in children in eastern Kentucky[2]). However, although *Strongyloides* is mainly restricted to tropical and subtropical regions, subclinical infection can be present many years after leaving an endemic area. Also, *Strongyloides* is always a potentially dangerous pathogen, so it is vitally important that medical technologists in developed countries should be able to recognize its presence.

Morphology

Only females are parasites of man and are very small, threadlike, transparent worms with a pointed tail which are 2.0–2.2 mm in length and between 0.04 and 0.06 mm in width. The oesophagus occupies the anterior third of the body and the vulva opens a third of the way from the anterior end. The ovaries, oviducts and uteri are paired and there are usually about 10 parthenogenetically produced eggs in each uterus.

Strongyloides can also maintain a free-living cycle in the soil, in which case morphologically distinct females and males are found. The females are shorter and stouter than the parasitic forms with a shorter muscular oesophagus whilst the males measure 0.7 × 0.04 mm with a pointed tail and two copulatory spicules.

Life cycle (Figure 5.1)

Strongyloides has a complex life cycle in that it can live as a parasite or as a free-living organism.

The parasitic females bury themselves in the mucosa of the small intestine and eggs are laid in the mucosa and submucosa (Figure 5.2). The thin-shelled eggs measuring 50–60 μm by 30–35 μm develop and hatch into first-stage larvae within the tissues of the mucosa. These larvae reach the intestinal lumen and pass out in the faeces; they measure about 0.25 mm and are said to be 'rhabditiform' because their muscular oesophagus with its enlarged posterior portion resembles that of a particular free-living nematode (*Rhabditis*). If the faeces are deposited on soil, the larvae feed on bacteria and moult twice resulting in the non-feeding infective third-stage. These infective larvae measure 0.55 × 0.02 mm and have a triradiate tip to the tail; unlike hookworm larvae there is no sheath from the second stage onwards. These larvae can survive about two weeks in the soil but are unable to exist at temperatures below 8 °C. They are also killed by drying or by excessive moisture.

When the larvae come into contact with skin, they penetrate it and initially enter the small cutaneous blood vessels before reaching the lungs. They migrate into the alveoli, moult twice, and then as immature adults pass up the bronchi and trachea and are swallowed down the oesophagus and ultimately enter the small intestine where they burrow into its mucosa (principally of the duodenum and jejunum). About 17 days after penetration the female worms begin to lay

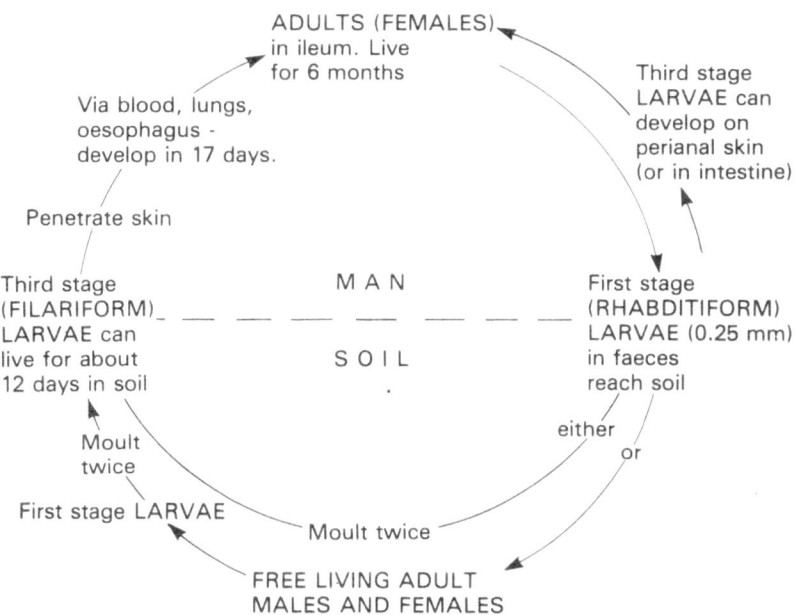

ADULTS (FEMALES) in ileum. Live for 6 months

Third stage LARVAE can develop on perianal skin (or in intestine)

Via blood, lungs, oesophagus - develop in 17 days.

Penetrate skin

M A N

Third stage (FILARIFORM) LARVAE can live for about 12 days in soil

S O I L

First stage (RHABDITIFORM) LARVAE (0.25 mm) in faeces reach soil

Moult twice

First stage LARVAE

either

or

Moult twice

FREE LIVING ADULT MALES AND FEMALES

Figure 5.1 *Strongyloides* life cycle

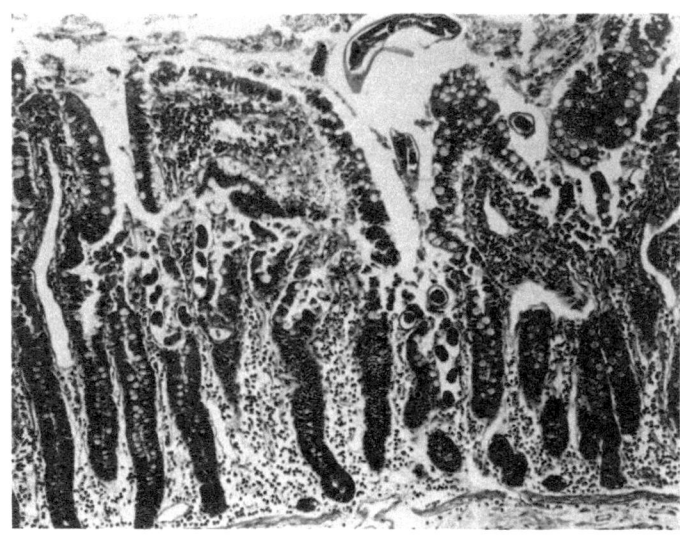

Figure 5.2 *Strongyloides* in small intestine

their parthenogenetically-produced eggs.

Auto-infection can occur if first-stage larvae passing out in faeces are deposited on the perianal skin and develop to the infective stage. In this way infection can persist for many years after a person has left an endemic area. Indiscriminate smearing of excrement, as may occur in mental institutions or amongst young children, is the most likely mode of transmission in developed countries.

In some instances, particularly in severely ill patients, first-stage larvae may develop into infective forms and penetrate the wall of the large bowel without reaching the exterior at all.

Rarely, when the hosts' cell-mediated defences are deficient, larvae may be found in almost all organs of the body and may even appear in the sputum.

Mode of transmission

The infective filariform larvae which live on the soil and in damp grass in warm countries can penetrate directly through unbroken skin, usually of the feet or lower legs.

Prevention

The sanitary disposal of faeces and the wearing of shoes means that this infection is not common in developed countries. Also, the larvae in the soil are unable to survive below 8 °C so that infection is likely to be very seasonal in temperate climates.

However, even in developed countries under conditions where indiscriminate defaecation occurs, strongyloidiasis may present an important clinical problem. Such a situation has been reported from a home for mentally retarded children in New York, where 17% of the inmates were infected in 1962 (although intensive chemotherapy had reduced this figure to 3% by 1970[3]).

In tropical countries the larvae are typically found in warm, shaded, moist areas such as coffee, cocoa and banana plantations.

Pathology

Penetration of the skin by the infective larvae may cause a form of erythematous pruritus known as ground itch, followed by blisters or papules associated with secondary bacterial infection caused by scratching. Larvae migrating through the lungs can also cause a diffuse pneumonitis similar to Loeffler's syndrome in ascariasis (see page 94).

The most important pathological effects are associated with the presence of adult females, larvae and eggs in the crypts of the duodenum and jejunum. The traumatic and irritating action of the parasites causes superficial damage to the mucosa resulting in eosinophil and mononuclear cell infiltration and increased secretory activity of the epithelium, producing a catarrhal enteritis. There may be numerous superficial small haemorrhages.

When auto-infection occurs, parasites penetrate more deeply into the sub-mucosa which then becomes oedematous, so that larvae may even gain access to lymphatics or small blood vessels.

In severe infections the villi become enlarged and the mucosa atrophies, a similar picture to that seen in tropical sprue. The parasites cause ulcers (up to 1 cm) in the atrophic mucosa of the small intestine and of the colon, leading to inflammatory infiltration, oedema, granuloma formation, and eventually fibrosis. Secondary bacterial invasion of the ulcers accentuates the inflammatory response. It is probable that decreased mobility of the intestine allows first-stage larvae to develop to the infective third-stage forms before being passed out of the anus. Cases of paralytic ileus have also been recorded as a complication[4].

Hyperinfection by filariform larvae is characterized by lesions in the colon, lymph nodes, lungs, liver and other organs in addition to the small intestine, and occurs when the cell-mediated immune response is depressed. In developed countries this usually follows the replacement of lymphoid tissues by malignancies or treatment with corticosteroids, radiation and/or cytotoxic drugs[5-10]. The connection between disseminated strongyloidiasis and septicaemia has not been proved but it is a likely event.

Clinical features

The majority of people infected with *Strongyloides* appear to suffer no or few ill effects from their presence.

An itchy rash may be present a few days after infection, followed by mild respiratory symptoms such as chest pain and coughing (due to the migrating stages) but it is very likely that the parasite will be present for many years while the patient remains asymptomatic. However, unlike the majority of helminth infections, *Strongyloides* is able to multiply without external reinfection, so that an infected person can fall ill many years after leaving an endemic area: a fatal infection has been reported in a Jamaican after 12 years in England[4], and a case has been reported after 36 years. The factors responsible for the alteration in behaviour of the parasite are not known.

Moderate infections are characterized by intermittent diarrhoea, upper abdominal pain (mimicking peptic ulcer) and the eosinophilia typical of most helminth infections.

Severe infection is a rare event in well-nourished individuals but the outcome is often grave, even with adequate treatment. The manifestations are vomiting and acute abdominal pain, with passage of voluminous foul-smelling stools. A malabsorption syndrome develops with dehydration and electrolyte disturbance. Oedema may result from the protein loss[11] and paralytic ileus can produce abdominal distension.[12]

In clinically overt cases auto-infection always occurs and lesions are almost certain to be present in the gluteal region.

In patients with malignant lymphomas, or on immunosuppressive therapy, hyperinfection may result and larvae in the lungs can give rise to acute respiratory distress, while convulsive crises have been observed in patients with cerebral involvement. Such cases almost always end fatally, usually from dehydration or from secondary bacterial infection[3-10].

It is thus important that, before any patient known to have resided in the tropics, even many years previously, is given immunosuppressive therapy, examination for *Strongyloides* should be made. Hyperinfection with *Strongyloides* should also be considered in any immigrant before laparotomy is performed.

Diagnosis

There is no pathognomonic clinical picture for strongyloidiasis, although an intermittent watery diarrhoea with mucus, in the presence of an eosinophilia, is suggestive. In clinically evident cases there are also likely to be the characteristic lesions in the gluteal region.

The only certain method of diagnosis is by identifying larvae in the faeces. *Strongyloides* is the only human nematode infection in which larvae rather than eggs are passed in faeces. These may be seen actively moving in a fresh faecal sample mixed with water and examined under the microscope. However, larvae may be scanty so that a concentration technique is necessary. The standard formol-ether method for helminth eggs and protozoal cysts can be used, as can Baermann filtration. In the latter method a stool sample is suspended in a filter funnel over water at about 45 °C and the larvae concentrate at the bottom of the funnel. Duodenal aspiration has also been advocated and a modification, in which a brushed nylon string is swallowed in a gelatin capsule and later withdrawn together with trapped larvae, can be very useful.

A charcoal culture method can be employed if no larvae can be found, but infection is suspected on clinical grounds. Five to ten grams of faeces are mixed with activated charcoal in a 10 cm diameter petri dish. The dish, dampened with distilled water, is covered and left for four days at 27 °C; any infective larvae are then removed from condensation drops on the lid with a small paintbrush.

Immunological methods of diagnosis are not very specific but this is normally not an important disadvantage in developed countries. Complement fixation or indirect haemagglutination, using antigen prepared from animal filarial worms, is fairly sensitive[13].

Treatment

The drug of choice at present is thiabendazole, which gives cure rates of 70–100%[14]. This is administered orally at a dose of 25 mg/kg body weight twice daily for two or three successive days; the treatment is repeated three weeks later since the agent is ineffective against eggs and first-stage larvae. Minor side effects, such as nausea and dizziness, are common. In severe cases intensive care with restoration of fluid albumin and electrolyte balance is essential. Secondary bacterial infection usually requires antibiotics. In cases of disseminated strongyloidiasis thiabendazole may not be effective[10, 12]. Mebendazole (Vermox) given at 100 mg twice daily for three days, irrespective of age or weight, has been successful in limited trials with children[15].

Enterobius vermicularis (the 'threadworm, pinworm or seatworm')

Geographical distribution

Enterobiasis is probably the most widespread and commonly occurring helminth infection of man and is found particularly in children. Infections are less common in tropical countries than in temperate climates where transmission is facilitated by the wearing of many clothes, and by overcrowding in schools, institutions or homes. It is likely that 15 million people are infected in the United Kingdom, 30 to 40 million in the United States and 30 million in Italy. However, although enterobiasis is typically regarded as a specifically childhood ailment, it is very much a family problem[16] and infection is by no means uncommon in adults.

Morphology

Threadworms are small fusiform nematodes, whitish in colour. The female dimensions are 8–12 mm by 0.3–0.5 mm. There is a long, pointed, tail and the body is usually distended by the bulk of eggs in the two uteri. The male is smaller (2–5 mm by 0.2 mm) with a ventrally curved tail and a single copulatory spicule. Expelled worms are often seen on the surface of the stool.

The oesophagus of both sexes is muscular with a posterior bulb, a characteristic of the Order Oxyurida. Lateral expansion of the cuticle down each side of the body (alae) make sections of worms easily recognizable.

Life cycle (Figure 5.3)

The adult worms live in the lumen of the caecum (Figure 5.4) and, if infection is heavy, the adjacent parts of the ascending colon and ileum.

After copulation, the male worms usually pass out of the host's anus. The females, laden with as many as 10 000 eggs, migrate through the anus, usually at night, and deposit the sticky eggs on the perianal and perineal skin. The translucent eggs measuring 54 by 24 μm are ovoid and flattened on one side. The ovum is usually partially developed by the time the egg is passed and an infective stage larva develops in 4–7 hours at 35 °C. Mature eggs remain viable

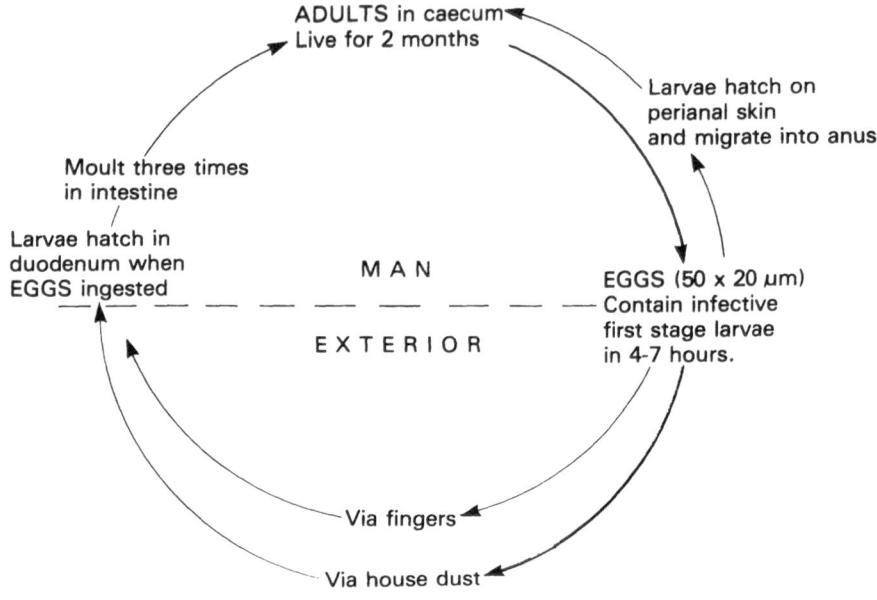

Figure 5.3   *Enterobius* life cycle

for 2–3 days at 22 °C and a relative humidity of 40%.

When ingested, first stage larvae (which measure 145 × 10 μm) hatch in the duodenum, moult three times, and reach maturity in two to five weeks. Adult worms live for only eight weeks but repeated reinfection often occurs.

Eggs sometime hatch on the perianal skin and larvae migrate back up the anus. Because of this process of retroinfection, infections can persist for months or years.

Mode of transmission

The most common mode of transmission, particularly in children, is from anus to hand to mouth. However, *Enterobius* eggs can survive for a few days in dirty clothes, soiled bed linen, or house dust, provided that they are kept cool and moist.

Because direct person-to-person transmission is so common, enterobiasis is primarily a familial and institutional infection.

Prevention

Following a course of chemotherapy, hands are washed thoroughly, underwear and bedclothes changed frequently, and bedrooms and lavatories vacuum cleaned.

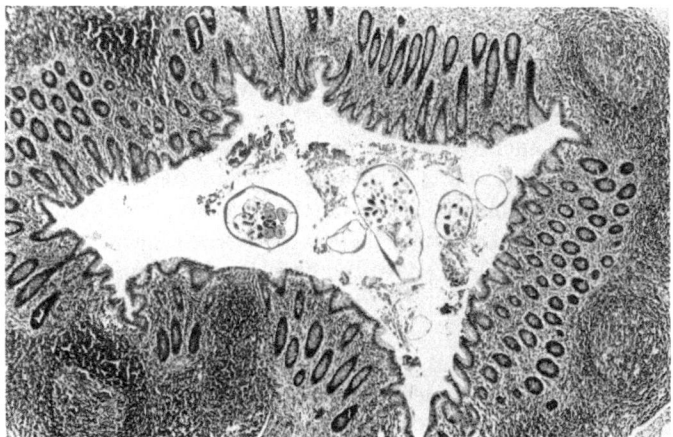

Figure 5.4 *Enterobius*: sections of adults in appendix, 0.3 mm in diameter

Clinical features

The adult worms attach to the intestinal mucosa and this can produce a mild catarrhal inflammation. However, there is no evidence that they can penetrate normal tissues.

The most common indication of *Enterobius* infection is itching in the perianal region. This follows the nocturnal migration of the female worms through the anus with the subsequent deposition of eggs on the perianal and perineal skin. The outer sticky, albuminous coat of the eggs can produce intense itching in sensitized individuals.

The consequent scratching can result in eczematous changes and secondary bacterial infection of the skin.

Many cases are symptomless but the most common symptom is the nighttime *pruritus ani* which can lead to loss of sleep. Because of the many possible causes for this condition it is likely that many cases in adults remain undiagnosed. Other effects which have been attributed to threadworms, such as anorexia, weight loss, fits, masturbation and nail biting, are dubious, although there is evidence for urinary tract infection and bedwetting in young girls[17, 18]. For girls, ova shed in the lower genital tract can produce vaginitis and are a common cause of *pruritus vulvae*. Migration of worms into the female genital tract can lead to vaginitis, endometritis and occasionally salpingitis or intra-abdominal inflammation[19].

It is likely that very rarely the presence of large number of adult worms in the appendix can lead to appendicitis[20], and a few cases of worms in the peritoneal cavity[21] or worms causing granulomas in the liver[20] have been reported.

There is usually a low grade eosinophilia of up to 12%.

Diagnosis

Eggs are only rarely found in the faeces but stick to the perianal skin and can be picked up using a swab technique with sticky tape, (Sellotape, or Scotch tape). An 8 cm length of tape, folded sticky side out over a microscope slide, is pressed firmly against each side of the perianal skin. The tape is then pressed sticky side down onto the slide and a drop of xylene run under it to increase transparency. The characteristic eggs, containing a larva and flattened on one side, can be easily recognized under the low power of a microscope.

A simple but effective sticky polythene envelope is manufactured in Japan and is distributed free to general practitioners; this obviates the need for slides or xylene.

Ideally the swab should be taken first thing in the morning and, if negative, repeated several times. A single test will detect about 50% of infections.

Active adult worms are sometimes observed on the surface of the stool or around the anus at night and should be preserved in alcohol for transport to the laboratory.

Treatment

There are now a number of well tolerated drugs (listed below) which result in a high cure rate. However, whichever drug is selected, it is advisable to treat the entire family or group to prevent immediate reinfection[22].

1. Mebendazole (Vermox). This is a broad spectrum antihelminthic and is given as a single oral dose of 100 mg for all ages[15].
2. Piperazine adipate (Antepar). Piperazine has been in use for the last 20 years and has few side-effects. Its main disadvantage is that treatment needs to be maintained for several days. A typical regimen would be 9 mg piperazine/kg body weight daily for 7 days.
3. Pyrantel pamoate (Antiminth) is another broad-action compound which has a high rate of cure with few side effects. It is given as a single dose of 10 mg/kg body weight, repeated a fortnight later.
4. Pyrvinium pamoate (Vanquin). It has the disadvantage that it can stain underclothes red. It is administered as a single dose (5 mg/kg body weight).
5. Levamisole (Ketrax) is another effective drug which can be given as a single dose (2.5 mg per kg body weight).

Ascaris lumbricoides ('roundworm')

Geographical distribution

Ascariasis is cosmopolitan in distribution although most commonly found in those humid tropical countries which have a low standard of hygiene. It is probable that about one quarter of the world's population is infected. Infection is said not to be common in most developed countries although recent estimates of infection in children are 75% in Italy, 21% in Spain, 18–40% in northern France and 20–50% in eastern Kentucky. In a survey of 6 million people in Japan in 1964, 65% were found to be passing *Ascaris* eggs.

In developed countries, infection is usually confined to pockets in rural areas where sewage systems are inadequate, and is markedly familial. For instance a 10% infection rate was found in children in southern Virginia and 82% of the parents of infected children were also passing eggs[23].

Morphology

These are large fusiform nematodes, creamy-white in colour. The females measure 20–40 cm by 0.3–0.6 cm, and the males 15–30 by 2–4 mm with a ventrally curved tail and two copulatory spicules. The size of both sexes is appreciably smaller in heavy infections.

Life cycle (Figure 5.5)

Each fertilized female worm produces about 200 000 eggs daily which are passed out in the faeces of the host. The egg measures 45–75 μm by 35–50 μm, and contains an unsegmented ovum when passed. The egg-shell has a coarsely mammilated outer sticky coat, stained brown by bile salts. In moist

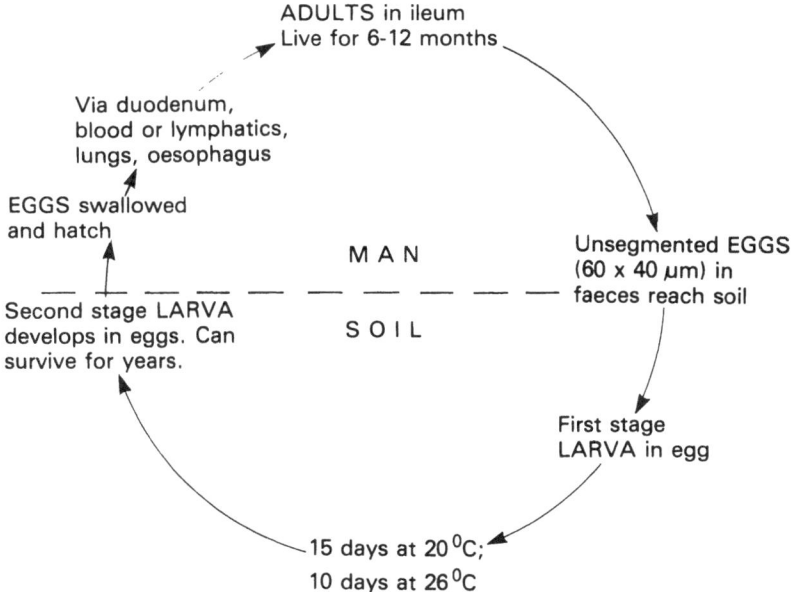

Figure 5.5 *Ascaris* life cycle

soil or in water at 20–30 °C, the ova within the egg take 10–15 days to develop to the infective second stage larvae. The larvae inside the eggs can survive for many years in temperate climates, although the ova will not develop at temperatures below 18 °C. When infective eggs are ingested, probably in salad vegetables, the larvae hatch out in the duodenum and begin an extraordinary somatic migration before settling down as responsible adults in the small intestine to the taxing business of egg production. The larvae penetrate the duodenal wall and enter the lymphatics or veins, migrate through the liver and heart, to reach the lungs in about four days. The larvae moult twice in the lungs, penetrate the alveolae, ascend the trachea and pass down the oesophagus, to reach the duodenum ten days later (Figure 5.6). They develop into adult males and females and eggs are passed in the faeces 60–75 days after the original ingestion of eggs. The adult lifespan is between six and twelve months.

Diagnosis

In the great majority of cases there is no problem in diagnosing infection since numerous eggs are passed in the faeces. In an autopsy study, eggs were always found if three or more adult female worms were present[24]. About 15% of all eggs are infertile and these are not so easily recognizable as they are larger and thinner (90 × 40 μm), have a thin shell and do not contain a discrete ovum.

Adult *Ascaris* can often be diagnosed radiologically as filling defects in straight X-rays of the abdomen. The intestine of the worm may be visible as a white line. Intravenous cholangiography is helpful in cases of biliary ascariasis[25,26].

Clinical diagnosis is not usually made, although if the early pulmonary symptoms occur, the accompanying eosinophilia is very suggestive.

Treatment

There are many new compounds which will effectively expel adult *Ascaris*, and they are listed below:

1. Mebendazole (Vermox) is given over three days in divided doses at 200 mg per kg body weight daily. This compound has the advantage that it is also active against most other helminth parasites such as *Enterobius*, *Trichuris* and hookworms.
2. Levamisole (Ketrax) at a dosage of 5 mg per kg body weight is very effective.
3. Pyrantel pamoate (Antiminth) is given at a dosage of 2.5–10 mg per kg body weight.
4. Piperazine salts (Antepar) can be given as a single dose of 80 mg per kg body weight and have been in use for the last 25 years.

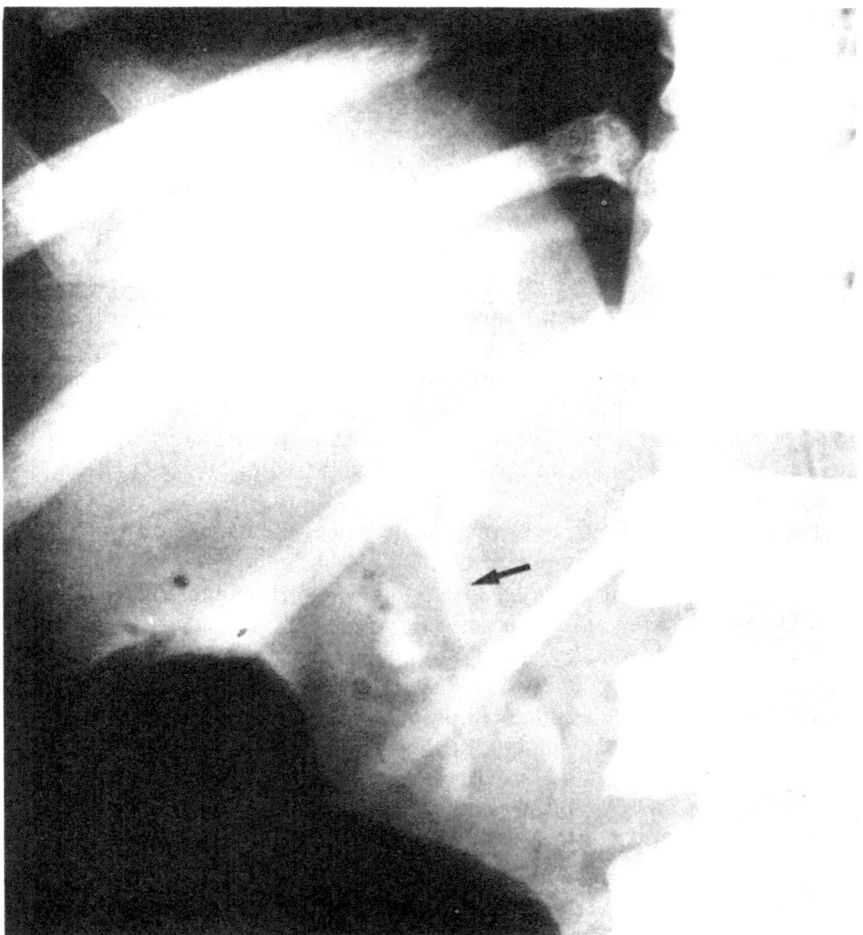

Figure 5.6 Dilated common bile duct containing *Ascaris* worm (translucent band). Behind lower end of common bile duct some of the contrast media is being excreted by the kidney (normal)

Mode of transmission

Eggs containing infective larvae are usually ingested on salad vegetables. Eggs are destroyed or removed by modern sewage treatment but ova can remain viable for many months in cesspits[27].

Clinical features

Almost all infections picked up in developed countries are light and likely to result in no symptoms at all. It has been estimated that, of about 1.3 million cases of *Ascaris* infection in the United States, the parasite could be implicated as a cause of death in only 38[28].

Larvae in the lungs often cause pneumonitis with a cough, wheezing and dyspnoea accompanied by eosinophilia, beginning about 5 days after infection and lasting almost two weeks (Loeffler's syndrome).

Biliary ascariasis is characterized by a sudden colicky pain in the upper right quadrant with vomiting and, where the worms are trapped, jaundice and abnormal liver function. In the latter case surgery is necessary but otherwise medical treatment should be adequate[26].

The major danger of complications in developed countries follows measures which increase the restlessness of the worms. This may be caused by various drugs, perhaps by peppery food and, in particular, following abdominal surgery. The possibility of a heavy *Ascaris* infection should be borne in mind before carrying out intestinal surgery in any patient who has come from the tropics. Increasing affluence in oil-rich countries in particular is resulting in many more possibly infected patients seeking treatment in hospitals in developed countries.

In the tropics, where infections may be very heavy, intestinal obstruction is the most common complication. Obstruction may be completely mechanical in nature but may be due to intestinal spasm following irritation of sensory receptors in the ileum. Rarely, there may be intussusception or volvulus and worms may penetrate the appendix giving symptoms of acute appendicitis. Intestinal obstruction was found in 66% of 528 acute emergencies caused by *Ascaris* over a 13-year period in children (mostly 4–8 year olds) in South Africa[26], which in turn constituted about 12% of all intestinal emergencies. In such cases pain may recur over a period of weeks or months and there is often a history of worms having been passed in the vomit or faeces.

Anisakis

The cause of eosinophilic granulomas of the small intestine and stomach found in Holland and in Japan was first identified as a helminth parasite, *Anisakis simplex*, in Holland in 1960[29]. In both countries raw marine fish is popular thus the name of 'herring worm disease' was given to the condition transmitted by this foodstuff. The living larvae ingested in fish penetrate the mucosa of the alimentary canal causing small haemorrhages and necrosis, leading to tumour-like granulomas. A blood eosinophilia of 3–30% is found. In Holland these lesions are usually in the intestine and in Japan in the stomach. Symptoms of abdominal pain, nausea and vomiting closely simulate peptic ulcer or acute appendicitis. In fact, the correct diagnosis is usually only made by the pathologist after surgery has been carried out. In some patients infection follows a chronic course with episodes of abdominal pain persisting for years. The larvae do not mature in man; the natural final hosts are marine fish-eating mammals.

The condition appears to have vanished from Holland in the last few years, probably because all fish are now deep-frozen and the so-called 'green' herrings are banned. Larvae are all dead in 24 h at −17 °C but can survive for over a week at −5 °C. A few cases have been reported from other western countries—Denmark, England, West Germany, United States—and it is possible that other cases have not been diagnosed.

Necator americanus ('New World hookworm') and *Ancylostoma duodenale* ('Old World hookworm')

Geographical distribution

There are two parasite species which cause hookworm infection in man and both are confined mostly to the tropics and subtropics. Both species are common in Africa, Asia and South America, and occur in Northern Australia, Japan and Portugal. *Necator* is also found in the southern United States and the West Indies, and *Ancylostoma* in Italy and the North African littoral. Hookworm is essentially a rural disease, occurring principally where there is high rainfall and shade, low standards of hygiene, and where the people walk barefoot.

Hookworm was formerly an important disease in the southern United States but was dramatically reduced by a campaign of treatment, public health measures and education, involving one million people in 11 states, between 1910–1914. However, there are still rural areas where infection is common in children, for example a 12% infection rate was found in southern Georgia[30] and 14.8% in Kentucky[31]. In Great Britain transmission is possible when there is a good summer, but in all northern Europe infection is normally found only in immigrants.

Morphology

Hookworms are small fusiform nematodes, greyish-white in colour, with the head bent back dorsally. There is a large buccal capsule, which has either two pairs of teeth (*A. duodenale*) or a pair of ventral cutting plates (*N. americanus*). *Ancylostoma* males measure about 10 by 0.5 mm, those of *Necator* 8 by 0.3 mm; the females of each species are slightly larger. The males have a membranous enlargement at the posterior end which is used in copulation, and known as a caudal bursa. This differs in structure slightly in the two species.

Life cycle (Figure 5.7)

The adult worms live in the small intestine and the females pass eggs into the lumen; about 10 000 per worm per 24 hours in the case of *Necator* and double that number for *Ancylostoma*. The thin-shelled eggs of the two types are

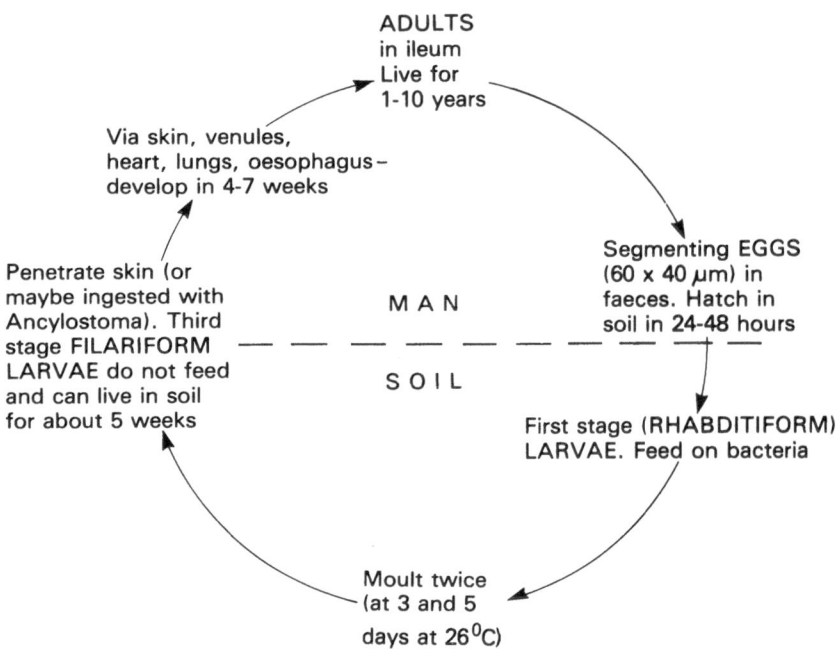

Figure 5.7   Hookworms life cycle

morphologically identical and measure 60 by 40 μm. The ovum is unsegmented when laid but is usually at the 4- or 8-celled stage when passed in
the faeces. If the faeces are deposited on soil, a first-stage rhabditiform larva
hatches from the egg within 24 hours. The larvae feed on organic matter and
bacteria in the soil and moult twice. The third-stage or filariform larvae retain
the cuticle of the previous moult and do not feed. They congregate in the top
few centimetres of soil or in the surface film of water on blades of grass. They
can survive for about four weeks in shaded, moist, sandy soil but on coming
into contact with human skin they can quickly penetrate it. There is evidence
that *Ancylostoma* larvae may also infect after ingestion, for example, on salad
vegetables.

After infecting through the skin or buccal mucosa, the larvae migrate via the
bloodstream to the heart and then to the lungs. The larvae grow in the lungs,
penetrate into the alveoli, ascend the bronchi and trachea, and are swallowed.
They complete their development and mature in the intestine. A process of
arrested development has been demonstrated for *Ancylostoma* infections in
India. Larvae contracted during the latter part of the monsoon season may
remain dormant in the body until the following year before developing into
adults[32]. It is possible, therefore, for infections to become patent many months
after a patient has left an endemic area.

Pathology

Hookworms attach to the mucosa of the small intestine and draw plugs of tissue into their buccal capsules. These are broken off and digested and the worms will then move on to new sites. This leads to numerous shallow lesions with consequent blood loss. The blood loss from this source has been estimated at 0.03 ml per 24 hours for an adult *Necator* and about three times that quantity for an *Ancylostoma*[33]. While such a blood loss can be very important in patients who have heavy worm loads and come from underdeveloped countries and hence have poor nutritional status, it is not of great significance in cases seen in the Western world. Similarly, severe hypoproteinaemia will only become apparent where there is already some degree of malnourishment.

Clinical features

A form of dermatitis known as ground itch often arises at the site of skin penetration by larvae. There may be an intense inflammatory response with blisters, papules and macules, perhaps complicated by secondary bacterial infection caused by scratching. The responses are usually more marked in reinfections.

Larval migration in the lungs occasionally causes coughing and wheezing, starting about one week after infection, and at this stage an eosinophilia is present.

In light infections, the adult worms in the gastrointestinal tract produce no symptoms at all, but in heavier infection there may be epigastric pain and tenderness simulating peptic ulcer.

In endemic areas high worm loads are sometimes associated with retardation of growth in children, severe anaemia perhaps with ensuing cardiac symptoms, and oedema.

Diagnosis

The most important method is by identifying eggs in the faeces. Any clinically important infection will have at least 2000 eggs per gram of faeces and these can be readily picked up in a direct faecal smear. For very light infections, as are usual in travellers from western countries who have visited the tropics, concentration methods such as the formol—ether technique may be required.

Techniques for determining which species of hookworm is present are given in standard textbooks (e.g. Muller, 1975[34]).

Treatment

Many of the broad spectrum antihelminthics mentioned in connection with *Enterobius* and *Ascaris*, such as mebendazole, levamisole and pyrantel pamoate, are also effective against hookworms. More specific drugs are bephenium (dosage: 5 g per day for 3 days) which is more effective against *Ancylostoma* than *Necator* and bitoscanate (adult dosage: 100 mg daily for 3 days). Repeated treatment may sometimes be required to totally eliminate all worms but is not clinically justified.

Thiabendazole, applied both as a topical 15% ointment for 3–4 days and at 25 mg/kg body weight twice daily for 2 days, is the best treatment for creeping eruption: this is caused by the infective larvae of non-human species of hookworms which creep around under the skin of man but fail to mature into adults.

Trichuris trichiura (the 'whipworm')

Geographical distribution

Trichuris is a cosmopolitan parasite but is particularly common in humid tropical climates. The best conditions for transmission are similar to those for *Ascaris* and the two parasites are often present in the same individual. Almost every individual may be infected where there is a low standard of sanitation in an endemic area and the eggs of *Trichuris* are probably the most common to be found in travellers returning from the tropics. It is estimated that there are at least 750 million cases in the world.

Transmission occurs in the southern United States and in southern Europe (e.g. an estimated 30% infection in Italy). In Great Britain infection is confined almost entirely to hospitals for mentally subnormal children in the south of England (with a 36% infection rate[35]). In the north the summer temperature is too low for eggs to develop to the infective stage.

Morphology

The female worm measures 30–50 mm in length and the male 30–45 mm; both sexes have a narrow thread-like anterior portion (about three-fifths of total length) and a wider posterior part. The non-muscular oesophagus occupies most of the anterior part with the reproductive organs in the thicker fleshy part. The anus is terminal. The caudal extremity of the male is coiled and it has a single spicule.

The adult worms are usually present in the caecum but may also occur in the appendix, rectum and upper colon, with the anterior portion embedded in the mucosa and the posterior hanging free.

Life cycle (Figure 5.8)

The female produces 2–10 000 eggs per day. The egg measures 52 by 22 μm and is barrel-shaped with transparent plug-like prominences at each end. The

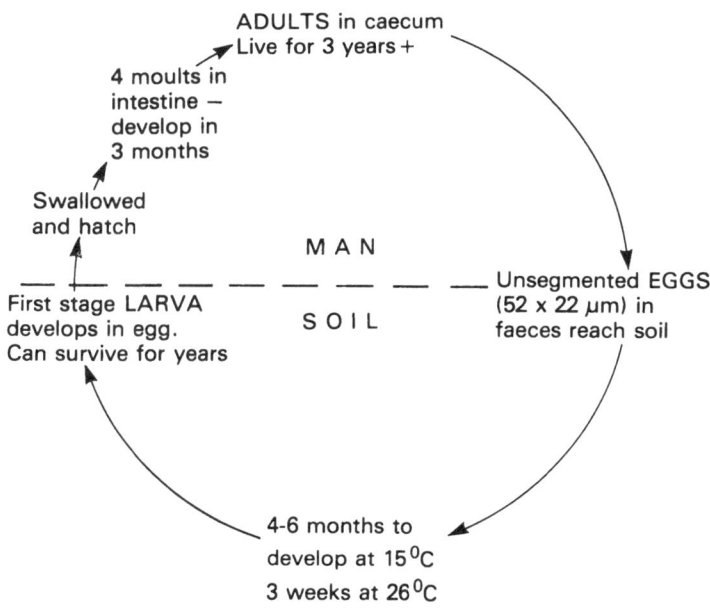

ADULTS in caecum
Live for 3 years +

4 moults in
intestine —
develop in
3 months

Swallowed
and hatch

M A N

First stage LARVA
develops in egg.
Can survive for years

S O I L

Unsegmented EGGS
(52 x 22 μm) in
faeces reach soil

4-6 months to
develop at 15°C
3 weeks at 26°C

Figure 5.8 *Trichuris* life cycle

ovum is unsegmented when laid and develops further in moist soil. They are infective in about three weeks in the tropics but take as many months at the summer temperatures found in southern England. Embryonated eggs are usually ingested on salad vegetables, although the habit of eating dirt (pica) is the usual mode of transmission in mental institutions in developed countries[36]. When the egg is swallowed, the contained first-stage larva hatches in the small intestine or colon and penetrates the mucosa where it develops further for about a week. After the usual four moults, the immature adult worms take up residence in the caecum and the female begins to produce eggs after two to three months. The adults normally live for about three years but can survive for at least ten.

Mode of transmission

This is solely by ingestion of eggs containing infective first-stage larvae. There is no multiplication within the human host so that for an infection to become heavier more eggs have to be ingested.

Prevention

Prevention consists of ensuring that all raw vegetables eaten are adequately washed in areas where transmission occurs.

Pathology

The adult worms live with the thin anterior portion of their bodies interlaced beneath the mucosa and cause small subepithelial haemorrhages.

In light infections significant lesions are not produced and the worms excite little cellular reaction. There may, however, be an eosinophilia of up to 15%.

Infection only becomes important when very large numbers of worms are present. When numbers approach 1000 (thought to correspond to about 30 000 eggs per gram of faeces), catarrhal inflammation, irritation and oedema, with plasma cell, eosinophil and polymorpholeukocyte infiltration of the mucosa, may be found. Diarrhoea is probably a result of impaired water reabsorption[36]. At sigmoidoscopy the colon appears hyperaemic and oedematous. Rectal prolapse has been described as a complication in very severe cases, possibly due to straining against the tangled mass of worms at defaecation or by the irritation of nerve endings with increased peristalsis.

Trichuris does suck blood but the amount is very small (about 0.005 ml per adult worm per day) and there will be a total loss of only 4 ml per day when 800 worms are present[37]; the effect is very unlikely ever to cause ill-effects in well-nourished individuals.

Clinical features

The light infections encountered in travellers returning from the tropics or found in individuals from endemic areas such as parts of southern Europe, parts of the southern United States and Queensland are invariably asymptomatic. Where symptoms are present in a lightly infected individual another cause should be sought, for instance amoebiasis (there is some evidence that the lesions caused by *Trichuris* can potentiate the pathogenic effect of various micro-organisms).

Very heavy infections with severe clinical symptoms seen sometimes in the tropics are almost always complicated by concomitant malnutrition. In developed countries such cases are seen only in inmates of mental institutions[36] and are characterized by chronic diarrhoea and abdominal pain. Appendicitis has been reported as a complication after obstruction of the lumen caused by numerous worms[38].

TISSUE NEMATODES

Trichinella spiralis (The 'trichina worm')

Geographical distribution

Trichinosis is cosmopolitan with a high prevalence in some temperate regions. Until recently infection was very important in the United States (particularly New York, New Jersey and Illinois) but the prevalence has fallen markedly in the last few years, with only 113 clinical cases reported for 1966–70, and 13 deaths. Trichinosis is also common in Eastern Europe with a prevalence of 3 to 4% in Poland and the adjoining areas of Russia (with a 1.1% overall prevalence in the latter). There are occasional outbreaks in Western Europe (particularly in Germany where raw pork products are popular) but infection is very uncommon in Great Britain and France.

However, infection still exists in animals in these countries and there were outbreaks in Liverpool and Glamorgan in 1953 with over 100 cases, and 26 soldiers who ate underdone pork after returning late from a training exercise in South Wales in 1969 also became infected[39]. The highest infection rates in the world are found in Eskimos (up to 50%) living in the Arctic north of Canada, Alaska and USSR. Clinical cases are also reported from South America, Asia and East Africa. There is no indigenous trichinosis in Australia.

Morphology

The minute thread-like adults (females 2.8 by 0.06 mm, males 1.1 by 0.03 mm) live partially embedded in the mucosa of the ileum and occur in carnivores, pigs and rats as well as in man. The oesophagus is non-muscular, unlike that of almost all other nematodes parasitizing man, but is surrounded by a column of glandular cells (the 'stichosome').

Life cycle (Figure 5.9)

Trichinella is unusual among the nematodes in that the same person acts as an intermediate and a final host. There are no free-living stages. The females in the small intestine produce first-stage larvae (measuring 100 by 5 μm) rather than eggs (ovoviviparity), and these are deposited in the mucosal tissues of the

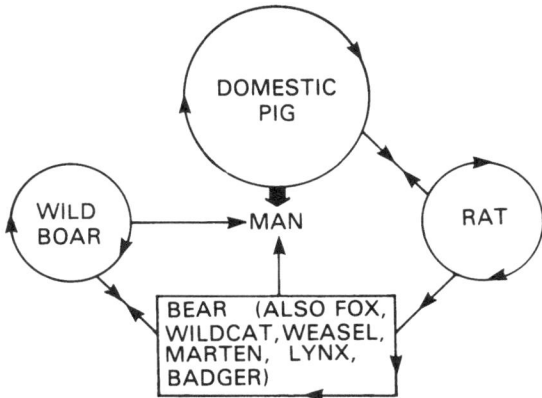

Figure 5.9 Cycle of *Trichinella* in temperate regions

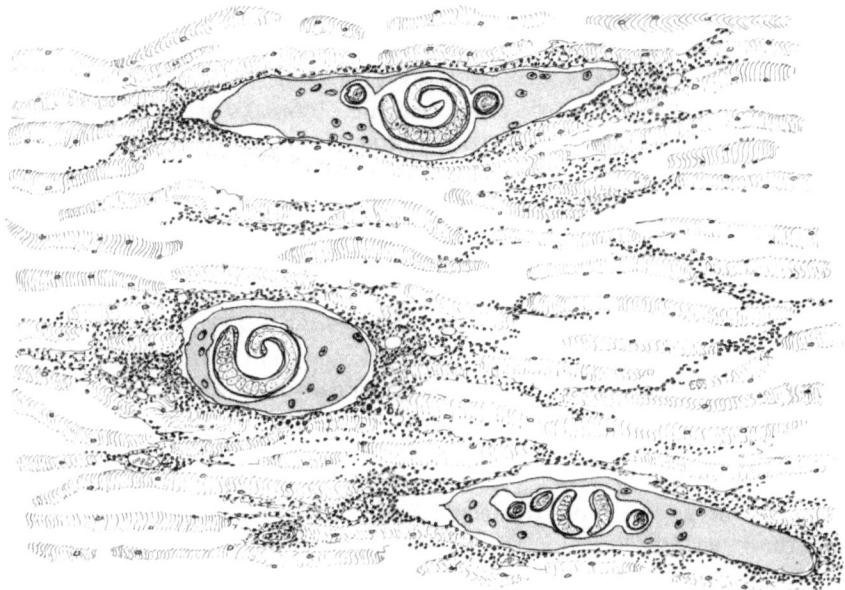

Figure 5.10 Diagram of section of skeletal muscle containing larvae of *Trichinella spiralis* in cysts. From a fatal case with severe myositis

ileum. The larvae are carried in the blood and lymphatics to all the skeletal muscles, where they penetrate the muscle cells (Figure 5.10). The larvae grow in days, and become surrounded by a collagenous capsule (measuring, on average, 0.4 by 0.26 mm). They are then infective to another host. Although the larvae can live in the muscle cysts for years, the wall of the cyst calcifies in a few months. The cysts are usually ingested by man in undercooked pork or pork products; the cyst walls are digested out in the stomach and the first-stage larvae which are released in the duodenum develop very quickly. They invade the mucosa and there moult four times; the immature adults have re-entered the lumen by 24 hours after fertilization and fertilized females appear after about 30 hours. Each female produces a total of 1200–2000 larvae and lives for only a few weeks. During the second and third weeks larvae may be present all over the body and some may be recovered from the faeces. However, after the third week larval migration diminishes.

Mode of transmission

Infection occurs in a wide range of animals, although in temperate regions the pig is of primary importance in infecting man. Human infection occurs particularly where home slaughtering is practised. In the Arctic and Africa wild animals only are involved and these strains of parasites will not easily infect

Table 5.2   The principal animal hosts of *Trichinella spiralis* in various geographical regions (those in capitals are eaten by man).

Region	Domestic cycle	Feral cycle
United States and Canada	PIG, rat, dog	BLACK AND BROWN BEAR, wild carnivores
Great Britain and Ireland	PIG, rat, cat	Fox
Western Europe	PIG, rat, cat, dog	WILD BOAR, carnivores, mustelids, rodents
Eastern Europe and USSR	PIG, rat, cat, dog, mouse	WILD BOAR, carnivores

pigs. Infections in Western countries also occur in hunters, usually contracted from bears in the United States and from wild boars in Europe (Table 5.2).

The cysts in muscle are very resistant to putrefaction and scavenging animals become infected by feeding on the dead bodies of other animals. Domestic pigs often become infected when pork scraps from other slaughtered animals are added to swill. Epidemics have occurred in the past, principally in Germany, Poland and the United States where raw pork products are popular. One of the most notorious outbreaks occurred in 1865 in the village of Hedersleben in Germany when 337 of the 2000 inhabitants became infected and 101 died.

Prevention and control

Uncooked pork products should be avoided and homemade pork sausages are a common cause of severe illness. In an outbreak in Ireland in 1968, 72% of patients admitted eating raw sausages[39].

The type of sausage may even be important, as the curious case of the bisected Penrith pig demonstrates. This infected pig was cut in two, half used for making sausages by one butcher and half by another in this small northern English town. However, all clinical cases of trichinosis occurred from the large type of sausage made by the first butcher and none from the small chipolata type sold by the other, which was presumably cooked more.

For those who would like an excuse for alcohol with their pork, experimental evidence in pigs and rats indicates that an Irish whiskey drunk at the same time provides a good degree of protection[40]. A detailed account of the control and surveillance measures, necessary to ensure that the risk of infected pork is minimized, is contained in Chapter 9.

Pathology

The adult worms cause small haemorrhages in the intestinal mucosa and some degree of hyperaemia occurs, giving rise to diarrhoea and abdominal pains. However, the important effect is due to the larvae in the muscles. The larvae cause myositis, with changes of swelling and oedema in the muscle fibres.

About 17 days after infection the remains of the muscle fibres appear more dense and there is a clear fluid area visible around each larva ('Nevinney's basophilic halo'), containing many nuclei. The outer translucent collagenous capsule is probably derived from the sarcolemma. There is an acute inflammatory response around the larvae, which become progressively encapsulated so that the oedema has subsided by the fifth week.

Larvae may also burrow into the heart or nervous tissues but do not encyst in these tissues. However, involvement of the heart or brain is potentially dangerous, since in both organs there is intense inflammation around each larva.

Clinical features

To a large extent the severity of symptoms depends on how many larvae are ingested. Luckily, the majority of infections are light and about 90% of patients have less than 10 larvae per gram of muscle. This level of infection causes eosinophilia (25–50%) about 12 days after ingestion of cysts, sometimes followed by mild muscle pains which resolve within a few months. In fact, many light infections remain undiagnosed during life and evidence of the parasite is only discovered at autopsy.

In heavy infections (over 100 cysts/g of muscle) clinical manifestations are varied and the disease is often misdiagnosed as typhoid or gastric flu. Typically there is marked eosinophilia (up to 80% with 4000 eosinophils per mm^3), high persistent fever, periorbital oedema, muscle tenderness, headache, tiredness, sore throat and gastrointestinal upsets, all reaching a maximum in the third or fourth week after infection. There may also be nervous system manifestations (including muscular paralysis), pulmonary complications (e.g. dyspnoea and bronchopneumonia) or cardiac involvement (dilatation and palpitations etc.). Muscular pain is usually severe and may last for several months. Cases with over 2000 larvae/g of muscle are almost always fatal, with death most likely to occur from exhaustion, pneumonia or cardiac failure between the fourth and eighth week of infection.

Diagnosis

Typical signs and symptoms are a high eosinophilia, puffiness of the eyes, generalized muscle pain, headache, fever and intestinal upsets. Diagnosis is usually easier when a group of people are infected together. Encysted larvae may be found in muscle biopsies by the fourth week of infection. A sample is taken from the biceps or gastrocnemius muscle and one half used for a direct squash and the other for the preparation of stained sections. However, larvae cannot always be found, particularly in early infections, and immunological methods of diagnosis are often necessary to confirm the clinical impression.

An intradermal test kit is commercially available (Wellcome Reagents) but it is not very sensitive in the early stages of infection; thereafter reactions often remain positive for years. This is a disadvantage in areas of decreasing incidence such as the United States (where there were an estimated 140 000 to 298 000 new infections in 1970 but only 109 reported clinical cases[41]) since it is important that any test should be able to distinguish between new and old cases. Complement fixation (CF), indirect fluorescent antibody (IFA), latex agglutination (LA), and bentonite flocculation (BF) tests are all commonly employed[41]. The IFA and new enzyme linked immunosorbent assay (ELISA) test can detect earlier infection than the others (10–20 days after infection)[42], while the LA and BF tests are the most convenient to carry out.

Treatment

Thiabendazole (Mintezol) is very effective against the migrating larvae when given orally at a dosage of 50 mg/kg body weight per day for 5 to 7 days, but is less effective against the encapsulated forms. Pyrantel pamoate (10 mg/kg body weight) and tetramisole (Ketrax) (2–5 mg/kg body weight) act only against the adult forms in the intestine and early diagnosis is essential if they are to act before the female worms have released many larvae. Large doses of corticosteroids (e.g. 25 mg of cortisone, four times daily, for four to five weeks) attenuate the allergic responses to the muscle phase and must be given when there are neurological complications. However, adult worms must be removed before steroid therapy as these compounds inhibit their expulsion.

VISCERAL *LARVA MIGRANS*

This general term is used to denote helminths in man which do not reach maturity but wander in the deeper organs of the body; occasionally they can be the cause of serious disease.

Toxocara

In the western world the most important example is the common ascaris of the dog (*Toxocara canis*) and possibly also *Toxascaris leonina* and the ascaris of the cat (*Toxocara cati*). The morphology and life cycle of these parasites is considered in Chapter 8 and the treatment here is confined to that of human infection.

Mode of transmission to man

Human infection follows the ingestion of infective eggs containing second stage larvae, on soil or salad vegetables which are contaminated by dog faeces. Larvae hatch from the eggs in the intestine, penetrate its wall, and reach the lungs and liver via the bloodstream. There is a similarity to *Ascaris* in the route of

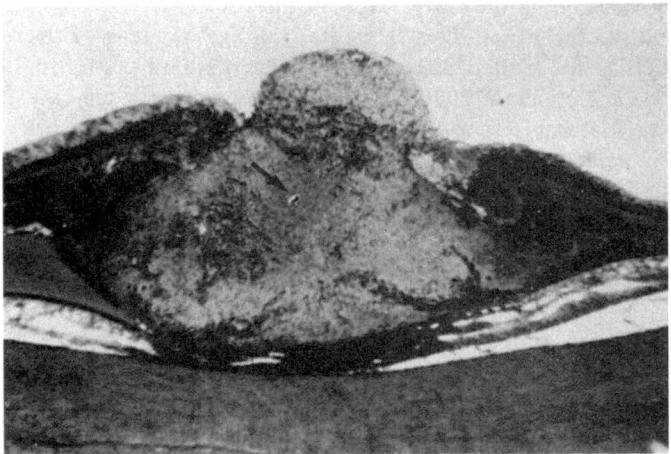

Figure 5.11   *Toxocara* in eye (low power)

migration but the larvae of *Toxocara* do not mature in man and being thinner can sometimes pass through the sinusoids and disperse to the kidneys, brain or eyes (Figures 5.11 and 5.12).

Pathology

The second stage larvae cause haemorrhages in the liver cells when they leave the sinusoids and burrow through the liver tissues. They elicit a strong immune response and the larvae become surrounded by an inflammatory response. An eosinophilic microabscess forms, comprising layers of eosinophils, plasma cells, lymphocytes and histiocytic cells. Later, fibrosis and possibly calcification occur. In tissue sections it is often impossible to identify portions of larvae in the centre of the host reaction, although if present, the characteristic lateral ridges allow positive identification.

Macroscopically, numerous white toxocaral granulomas are evident in the portal tracts, each measuring 3–4 mm in diameter. The granulomatous reaction which results from larvae reaching the eye may result in endophthalmitis and the formation of a granulomatous retinitis. These lesions are unilateral and larvae near the macula in young children have led to disturbance of vision[44]. In the past they have been erroneously diagnosed as retinoblastomas and the eye removed.

Clinical features

Overt disease is very rare and occurs principally in young children who have been playing in areas contaminated by dog faeces and have ingested eggs in

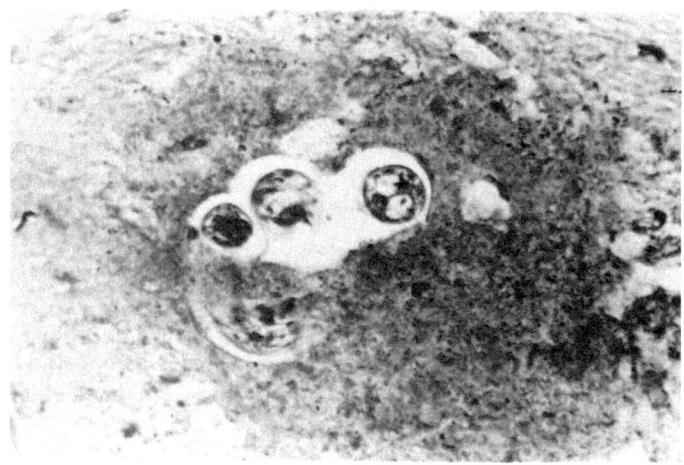

Figure 5.12   Toxocariasis of the eye. Larva in section (high power)

soil. Municipal sandpits, often used as dog's lavatories, probably provide suitable transmission conditions.

The incubation period is not clearly defined but is probably measured in days. Typical clinical features are tender hepatomegaly, hypereosinophilia (up to 60%) lasting for many months, and raised gammaglobulins. These manifestations may be preceded by respiratory symptoms such as cough, dyspnoea and bronchospasm, with a fever and perhaps allergic skin reactions. Larvae in the brain can result in epilepsy[45].

Diagnosis

In the past many cases have been diagnosed by accident following the examination of biopsy specimens for other reasons. Liver biopsy has been advocated but it is extremely unlikely that a portion of a larva will be present in a specimen taken at random. Laparoscopy is feasible; the granulomas surrounding trapped larvae appear as pale nodules on the surface of the liver and a biopsy specimen of one of these can be sectioned.

Clinically, long-lasting tender hepatomegaly, hypereosinophilia and raised gammaglobulin levels are suggestive but the important differential diagnosis is infection with the sheep liver fluke *Fasciola* (page 126).

Skin tests and most serological tests usually cross-react with *Ascaris* infections[44] but the indirect fluorescent antibody technique (IFAT) shows great promise using soluble antigens purified by affinity chromatography[46], and the enzyme-linked immunosorbent assay (ELISA) also appears to be species-specific.

Treatment

It is difficult to test the efficacy of treatment since it is based entirely on the amelioration of symptoms, and there is often spontaneous improvement in any case.

Diethylcarbamazine given orally at a dosage of 9 mg per kg body weight daily in three divided doses for 21 days has proved efficacious in a few cases[46] as has thiabendazole[47]. Corticosteroids have been used to combat the rare cases of acute respiratory distress[48].

In recent years a number of lurid articles proclaiming the dangers to children of keeping pets have appeared in the popular press of many western countries. These reports have tended to exaggerate greatly the dangers from toxocariasis; symptomatic cases are in fact very rare. However, this is perhaps no bad thing if such stories will help to reduce the quantity of dog excrement which befouls so many cities.

NEMATODE INFECTIONS CONFINED TO THE TROPICS

Most of the nematode infections which have been considered already, such as *Strongyloides*, *Ascaris*, *Trichuris* and the hookworms, are very much more common in tropical than in temperate regions. This, however, is not dictated entirely by climate but is also affected by lower standards of hygiene. There are also some other important nematode infections of man where transmission is possible only in warm countries. Nowadays, with holidays being taken ever further afield, even these infections may be not uncommonly found in returning travellers seen at general practice or in hospitals in the Western world.

The most important group of nematode infections in man confined entirely to the tropics and subtropics are the filariae. These are all tissue dwelling parasites, which are transmitted by blood feeding insects. Their important features are shown in Table 5.3.

Wuchereria and the closely related *Brugia* are an important cause of disease in the tropics but it is unlikely that any traveller to an endemic region will become infected. If they should, it is even more unlikely that microfilariae will appear in the peripheral blood. During the Second World War, over ten thousand American servicemen were infected with *W. bancrofti* in the south western Pacific and Samoa but less than 20 had a fleeting microfilaraemia[50]. Similar experiences occurred with French servicemen in Indochina in the 1950s.

If an adult from a non-endemic area becomes infected, there may be recurring attacks of acute lymphangitis with tender swollen lymph glands accompanied by mild pyrexia, headache and nausea beginning about 8–12 months later. In males there may also be inflammation of the scrotum, perhaps leading to hydrocoele, but the grotesque and disfiguring sequel of elephantiasis does not occur under such circumstances.

Table 5.3 Features of the filariae

Parasite	Geographical distribution	Site of adult	Site of microfilariae	Vector	Associated pathology
Wuchereria bancrofti	Africa, Asia South America Pacific	Lymphatics	Bood (sheathed)	Mosquitoes	Lymphangitis, hydrocoele, elephantiasis
Brugia malayi	South East Asia	Lymphatics	Blood (sheathed)	Mosquitoes	Lymphangitis, elephantiasis
Loa loa	West and Central Africa	Subcutaneous	Blood (sheathed)	Chrysops	Fugitive swellings
Mansonella ozzardi	South America, West Indies	Peritoneal cavity	Blood (unsheathed)	Culicoides	None
Dipetalonema perstans	Africa, South America	Peritoneal cavity	Blood (unsheathed)	Culicoides	None
D. streptocerca	West Africa	Subcutaneous	Skin (unsheathed)	Culicoides	Minor skin changes
Onchocerca volvulus	Africa, Yemen, Central and South America	Subcutaneous	Skin (unsheathed)	Simulium	Skin changes, blindness
Dirofilaria spp.	Africa, Asia, Americas	Subcutaneous, lungs, subconjunctiva	Not found in man	Mosquitoes	Abscess

Microfilariae of *Loa loa, Dipetalonema perstans* or *Mansonella ozzardi* are not uncommonly found in the blood of expatriates who have lived for some time in an endemic area. The microfilaraemia is usually low and infections are asymptomatic. Loiasis is clinically the most important; in 45 Europeans infected in West Africa[51] fugitive swellings appeared without warning on the arms or legs 3–12 months after visiting the tropics, while in 29 of the patients worms also crossed the conjunctiva during the course of the infection. Diethylcarbamazine is an effective drug against both adults and microfilariae.

In the United States about 20 cases of infection with animal filariae (mostly species of *Dirofilaria* from the dog) have been reported[52].

Infection with *Onchocerca volvulus* is comparatively rare in travellers returning from tropical countries, mainly because it is confined to rural areas of West and Central Africa and Central America, which receive few visitors. However, it is a very common infection among the inhabitants of endemic regions near to rivers in which the vector blackfly (*Simulium* spp.) breeds. At present an internationally-aided seven country control scheme is being undertaken in the Volta river basin in West Africa.

The adult worms live subcutaneously in tangled masses, usually in palpable nodules at pressure points. However, it is the microfilariae, present in the skin rather than in the blood, that are the principal pathological agents. About one year after infection the presence of the microfilariae results in pruritus with a persistent and itchy rash. Over the course of years the skin may become thickened and oedematous and this can be followed by atrophy of the skin with loss of elasticity, giving a prematurely aged appearance[53]. The most important sequel which might result from a heavy infection is blindness. Blindness occurs only in heavily infected persons who have lived in an endemic area for some years. It is usually caused by a sclerosing keratitis following reaction to the dead microfilariae in the cornea[54]. Diethylcarbamazine will kill microfilariae but needs to be given cautiously as it can give rise to intense itching.

References

1. Dancescu, P. (1968). Investigations on the intensity of the infection in a strongyloidiasis focus: the coal culture method. *Trans. Roy. Soc. Trop. Med. Hyg.*, **62,** 490
2. Fulmer, H. S. and Heumpfner, H. R. (1965). Intestinal helminths in Eastern Kentucky: a survey in rural counties. *Am. J. Trop. Med.*, **14,** 269
3. Seabury, J. H., Abadie, S. and Savoy, F. (1971). Pulmonary strongyloidiasis with lung abscess. Ineffectiveness of thiabendazole therapy. *Am. J. Trop. Med. Hyg.*, **20,** 209
4. Cookson, J. B., Montgomery, R. D., Morgan H. V. and Tudor R. W. (1972). Fatal paralytic ileus due to strongyloidiasis. *Br. Med. J.*, **4,** 771
5. Civantos, F. and Robinson, M. J. (1969). Fatal strongyloidiasis following corticosteroid therapy. *Am. J. Dig. Dis.*, **14,** 543
6. Cruz, T., Reboucas, G. and Rocha, H. (1966). Fatal strongyloidiasis in patients receiving corticosteroids. *N. Engl. J. Med.*, **275,** 1093
7. Dwork, K. G., Jaffe, J. R. and Lieberman, H. D. (1975). Strongyloidiasis with massive hyperinfection. *N.Y. State J. Med.*, **75,** 1230
8. Neefe, L. I., Pinilla, U., Garagus, V. F. and Bauer, H. (1973). Disseminated strongyloidiasis with cerebral involvement. A complication of corticosteroid therapy. *Am. J. Med.*, **55,** 832
9. Purtilo, D. T., Meyers, W. M. and Connor, D. H. (1974). Fatal strongyloidiasis in immunosuppressed patients. *Am. J. Med.*, **56,** 488
10. Rivera, E., Maldonado, N., Verlez-Garcia, E., Grillo, A. J. and Malaret, G. (1970). Hyperinfection syndrome with *Strongyloides stercoralis. Ann. Int. Med.*, **72,** 199
11. O'Brien, W. (1975). Intestinal malabsorption in acute infection with *Strongyloides stercoralis. Trans. Roy. Soc. Trop. Med. Hyg.*, **69,** 69
12. Royle, G., Fraser-Moodie, A. and Wansborough Jones M. (1974). Hyperinfection with *Strongyloides stercoralis* in Great Britain. *Br. J. Surg.*, **61,** 495
13. Kanan, S. R. and Rees, P. M. (1970). The diagnosis of strongyloidiasis with special reference to the value of the filarial complement fixation test as a screening test. *Trans. Roy. Soc. Trop. Med. Hyg.*, **64,** 246
14. Amir-Ahmadi, Braun, P., Neva, F. A., Gotlieb, L. S. and Zamcheck, N. (1968). Strongyloidiasis at the Boston City Hospital—Emphasis on gastrointestinal pathophysiology and successful therapy with thiabendazole. *Am. J. Dig. Dis.*, **13,** 959
15. Chongsuphajaisiddhi, T., Sabcharoen, A., Attanah, P., Panasoponkul, C. and Radomyos, P. (1978). Treatment of soil-transmitted nematode infections in children with mebendazole. *Ann. Trop. Med. Parasitol.*, **72,** 59
16. Miller, M. J., Krupp, I. M., Little, M. D. and Santos, C. (1974). Mebendazole. An effective anthelminthic for trichuriasis and enterobiasis. *J. Am. Med. Assoc.*, **230,** 1412
17. Sachdev, Y. V. and Howards, S. S. (1975). *Enterobius vermicularis* infestation and secondary enuresis. *J. Urol.*, **113,** 143
18. Simon, R. D. (1974). Pinworm infestation and urinary tract infection in young girls. *Am. J. Dis. Child.*, **128,** 21
19. McDonald, G. S. A. and Houritane, D. O'B. (1972). Ectopic *Enterobius vermicularis. Gut,* **13,** 621
20. Duran-Jorda, F. (1957). Appendicitis and enterobiasis in children. A histologic study of 691 appendixes. *Arch. Dis. Childh.*, **32,** 208
21. Little, M. D., Cuelloc, C. J. and d'Allessandra, A. (1973). Granuloma of the liver due to *Enterobius vermicularis.* Report of a case. *Am. J. Trop. Med. Hyg.*, **22,** 567
22. Matsen, J. M. and Turner, J. A. (1969). Reinfection in enterobiasis (pinworm infection). Simultaneous treatment of family members. *Am. J. Dis. Child.*, **4,** 576
23. Williams, D., Burke, G. and Hendley, J. O. (1974). Ascariasis: a family disease. *J. Pediatr.*, **84,** 853

24. Kannangara, D. W. N. (1975). A comparison of post mortem analysis of helminths with faecal egg counts. *Trans. Roy. Soc. Trop. Med. Hyg.*, **69**, 400

25. Cremin, B. J. and Fisher, R. M. (1976). Biliary ascariasis in children. *Am. J. Roentgenol., Radium Ther. Nucl. Med.*, **126**, 352

26. Louw, J. H. (1974). Biliary ascariasis in childhood. *S. Afr. J. Surg.*, **12**, 219

27. Shephard, M. R. N. (1971). The role of sewage treatment in the control of human helminthiasis. *Helminthol. Abstr.*, **40**, 1

28. Piggott, J., Hansberger, E. A. Jr. and Neafie, R. C. (1970). Human ascariasis. *Am. J. Clin. Pathol.*, **53**, 223

29. Jackson, G. J. (1975). The new disease status of human anisakiasis and north American cases: a review. *J. Milk Food Technol.*, **38**, 769

30. Martin, L. K. (1972). Hookworm in Georgia. *Am. J. Trop. Med. Hyg.*, **21**, 919

31. Gloor, R. F., Breyley, E. R. and Martiniz, I. G., (1970). Hookworm infection in a rural Kentucky county. *Am. J. Trop. Med. Hyg.*, **19**, 1007

32. Nawalinski, T. A. and Schad, G. A. (1974). Arrested development in *Ancylostoma duodenale*: course of self-induced infection in man. *Am. J. Trop. Med. Hyg.*, **23**, 895

33. Roche, M., and Layrisse, M. (1966). The nature and cause of 'hookworm anaemia'. *Am. J. Trop. Med. Hyg.*, **15**, 1030

34. Taylor, A. E. and Muller, R. (eds.) (1975). *Pathogenic Processes in Parasitic Infection.* (Oxford. British Society for Parasitology, Symposium 13)

35. Lynch, D. M., Green, E. A., McFadzean, J. A. and Pugh, I. M. (1972). *Trichuris trichiura* infestations in the United Kingdom and treatment with difetarsone. *Br. Med. J.*, **4**, 73

36. Mathan, V. I. and Baker, S. J. (1970). Whipworm disease. Intestinal structure and function of patients with severe *Trichuris trichiura* infestation. *Am. J. Dig. Dis.*, **15**, 913

37. Layrisse, M., Adarcedo, C. M. and Roche, M. (1967). Blood loss due to infection with *Trichuris trichiura. Am. J. Trop. Med. Hyg.*, **16**, 613

38. Haines, D. O., Buckley, J. J. C. and Pester, F. R. N. (1968). A cryptic infection of an appendix with the whipworm, *Trichuris trichiura* in Britain. *J. Helminthol.*, **42**, 289

39. Corridan, J. P. and Gray, J. J. (1969). Trichinosis in south-west Ireland. *Br. Med. J.*, **2**, 727

40. Campbell, W. C. (1977). Can alcoholic beverages provide protection against trichinosis? *Proc. Helminthol. Soc. Washington*, **44**, 120

41. Kagan, I. G. (1976). Serodiagnosis of trichinosis. In: S. Cohen and E. Sadun (eds) *Immunology of Parasitic Infections.* (Oxford: Blackwell)

42. Campbell, W. C. and Blair, L. S. (1974). Chemotherapy of *Trichinella spiralis* (a review). *Exp. Parasitol.*, **35**, 304

43. Duguid, I. M. (1971). Ocular infestation by *Toxocara. Br. J. Ophthalmol.*, **45**, 789

44. Woodruff, A. W. (1970). Toxocariasis. *Br. Med. J.* (Sept. 19), 663

45. Soulsby, E. J. L. (1976). In: S. Cohen and E. Sadun (eds). *Immunology of Parasitic Infections* (Oxford: Blackwell)

46. Wiseman, R. A., Woodruff, A. W. and Pettitt, L. E. (1971). The treatment of toxocaral infection: some experimental and clinical observations. *Trans. Roy. Soc. Trop. Med. Hyg.*, **65**, 591

47. Schartz, P. M., Glickman, T. L., Allain, D., Dykes, A. C. and Kagan, I. G. (1978). Clinical, serologic and epidemiologic studies of ocular toxocariasis. *4th Int. Congr. Parasitol. (Warsaw); Short Communications E.*, 97–98

48. Charleston, W. A. G. (1977). *Toxocara* and human health. *N.Z. Vet. J.*, **25**, 171

49. Beshear, J. R. and Hendley, J. O. (1973). Severe pulmonary involvement in visceral larval migrans. *Am. J. Dis. Child.*, **125**, 599

50. Edeson, J. F. B. (1972) Filariasis. *Br. Med. Bull.*, **26**, 60

51. Trent, S. (1963). Re-evaluation of World War II veterans with filariasis acquired in the South Pacific. *Am. J. Trop. Med. Hyg.*, **12**, 877

52. Connal, A. (1934). Calabar swellings. *W. Afr. Med. J.*, **7**, 113

53. Beaver, P. C. and Orihel, T. C. (1965). Human infection with filariae of animals in the United States. *Am. J. Trop. Med. Hyg.*, **14**, 1010

54. Buck, A. A. (ed.) (1974). *Onchocerciasis: Symptomatology, Pathology, Diagnosis.* (Geneva: World Health Organization)

55. Woodhouse, D. F. (1975). Tropical eye diseases in Britain. *Practitioner*, **214**, 646

Further Reading

Beaver, P. C. (1969). The nature of visceral larva migrans. *J. Parasitol.*, **53**, 3

Beaver, P. C. (1975). Biology of soil-transmitted helminths: the massive infection. *Health Lab. Sci.*, **12**, 116

Bhaskaran, C. S., Devi, E. S. and Rao, K. V. (1975). *Enterobius vermicularis* and vermiform appendix. *J. Ind. Med. Assoc.*, **64**, 334

Blumenthal, D. S. and Schulz, M. G. (1975). Incidence of intestinal obstruction in children infected with *Ascaris lumbricoides. Am. J. Trop. Med. Hyg.*, **24**, 801

Bradford, D. E., Richards, P. J., Warrington, T. G. A. L. and Webb, J. F. (1971). Trichinosis in Aldershot. *J. Roy. Army Med. Corps*, **117**, 117

Brown, R. C. and Girandrau, M. H. F. (1977). Transmammary passage of *Strongyloides* sp. larvae in the human host. *Am. J. Trop. Med. Hyg.*, **26**, 215

Buckley, J. J. C. and Pester, F. R. N. (1965). Hookworm infections acquired in Great Britain. *Br. Med. J.*, **2**, 106

Bustamente-Sarabia, J., Martuscelli, Q. A. and Tay, J. (1977). Ectopic ascariasis: report of a case with adult worms in the kidney. *Am. J. Trop. Med. Hyg.*, **26**, 568

Chabaud, A. G. (1974). *CIH Keys to the Nematode Parasites of Vertebrates.* No. 1 (Slough: Commonwealth Agricultural Bureaux)

Chu, W. G., Chen, P. M., Huang, C. C. and Hsu, C. T. (1972). Neonatal ascariasis. *J. Pediatr.*, **81**, 783

Collins, R. F. and Ivey, M. H. (1975). Specificity and sensitivity of skin test reactions to extracts of *Toxocara canis* and *Ascaris suum.* II. Homologous 48 hour passive cutaneous anaphylaxis tests with sera from infected guinea pigs, *Am. J. Trop. Med. Hyg.*, **24**, 460

Davis, A. (1973). *Drug Treatment in Intestinal Helminthiases.* (Geneva: World Health Organization)

Fangundes, L. A., Basuto, O. and Brentano, L. (1971). Strongyloidiasis: fatal complication of renal transplantation. *Lancet*, **ii**, 439

Fischer, R. M. and Cremin, B. J. (1970). Rectal bleeding due to *Trichuris. Br. J. Radiol.*, **43**, 214

Gilles, H. M. (1975). Hookworm infection and anaemia. *Trop. Doctor*, **5**, 51

Gupta, M. C., Basu, A. K. and Tandon, B. N. (1974). Gastrointestinal protein loss in hookworm and roundworm infections. *Am. J. Clin. Nutr.*, **27**, 1386

James, T. (1970). Ascarid abscess of the liver. A review of the evidence. *Med. Proc.*, **16**, 127

Kim, C. W. (ed.) (1974). *Trichinellosis.* (New York: Intext)

Lagundoye, S. B. (1972). Disordered small bowel pattern in ascariasis. *Trop. Geograph. Med.*, **24**, 226

Lee, E. L., Iynkaran, N., Grieve, A. W., Robinson, M. J. and Dissanaike, A. S. (1976). Therapeutic evaluation of oxantel pamoate in severe *Trichuris trichiura* infections. *Am. J. Trop. Med. Hyg.*, **25**, 563

Levine, N. D. (1968). *Nematode Parasites of Domestic Animals and Man.* (Minneapolis: Burgess)

Lintermans, J. P. (1975). Fatal peritonitis, an unusual complication of *Strongyloides stercoralis* infestation. *Clin. Pediatr.*, **14**, 974

Lotero, H., Tripathy, K. and Bolanos, O. (1974). Gastrointestinal blood loss in *Trichuris* infection. *Am. J. Trop. Med. Hyg.*, **23**, 1203

Lundy, M., Edkins, W. W., Kilpatrick, R., Goldsmith, E. F., Kosty, T. H. and Wolf, F. S. (1973). Hookworm disease—Alabama. Morbidity and mortality. *USD. Health Ed. Welf.*, **22**, 86

Marcial-Rojas, R. A. (ed.) (1971). *Pathology of Protozoal and Helminthic Diseases.* (Baltimore: Williams and Wilkins)

Marsden, P. D. (ed.) (1978). *Clinics in Gastroenterology*, Vol 7, no. 1. *Intestinal Parasites.* (Eastbourne: W. B. Saunders Co. Ltd.)

Martinez-Torres, C., Ojeda, A., Roche, M. and Layrisse, M. (1967). Hookworm infection and intestinal blood loss. *Trans. Roy. Soc. Trop. Med. Hyg.*, **61**, 373

Miller, M. J., Krupp, I. M., Little, M. D. and Santos, C. (1974). Mebendazole. An effective anthelminthic for trichuriasis and enterobiasis. *J. Am. Med. Assoc.*, **230**, 1412

Muller, R. (1975). *Worms and Disease: a Manual of Medical Helminthology.* (London: Wm. Heinemann Medical Books)

Poltera, A. A. (1972). Pulmonary strongyloidiasis. *Trans. Roy. Soc. Trop. Med. Hyg.*, **66**, 520

Reddy, C. R. R. M., Rao, D. V., Sarma, E. N. B. and Swamy, G. M. N. (1975). Granulomatous peritonitis due to *Ascaris lumbricoides* and its ova. *J. Trop. Med. Hyg.*, **78**, 146

Rim, H. J. and Lim, J. K. (1972). Treatment of enterobiasis and ascariasis with combantrin (Pyrantel pamoate). *Trans. Roy. Soc. Trop. Med. Hyg.*, **66**, 170

Scragg, J. N. and Proctor, E. M. (1977). Mebendazole in the treatment of severe symptomatic trichuriasis in children. *Am. J. Trop. Med. Hyg.*, **26**, 198

Spencer, H. (ed.) (1972). *Spezielle pathologische Anatomie*, Vol. 8, *Tropical Pathology*. (Berlin: Springer-Verlag)

Spillmann, R. K. (1975). Pulmonary ascariasis in tropical communities. *Am. J. Trop. Med. Hyg.*, **24**, 791

Sran, H. S., Dandia, S. D. and Dendse, A. K. (1973). Acute intestinal obstruction. A review of 504 cases. *J. Ind. Med. Assoc.*, **60**, 455

Turley, K. and Sherman, R. T. (1976). Biliary ascariasis. *Am. Surgeon*, **42**, 166

van Thiel, P. H. (1976). The present status of anisakiasis and its causitive worms. *Trop. Geograph. Med.*, **28**, 75

Yoeli, M., Most, H., Hammond, J. and Scheinesson, G. P. (1972). Parasitic infections in a closed community. *Trans. Roy. Soc. Trop. Med. Hyg.*, **66**, 764

Zimmerman, W. J. (1975). In W. T. Hubbert, W. F. McCulloch and P. R. Schnurrenberger (eds) *Diseases Transmitted from Animals to Man*, pp. 545–549. (Springfield, Illinois: Charles C. Thomas)

Zuidema, P., Rep, B. H. and Meuzelaar, H. L. C. (1972). Ancylostomiasis in Dutch servicemen returning from Surinam. *Trop. Geograph. Med.*, **24**, 68

6
Cestodes and Trematodes

D. R. SEATON

INTRODUCTION

Cestodes (tapeworms) and Trematodes (flukes) are two Classes of the Phylum Platyhelminthes. Tapeworms live in the intestines of vertebrates and their larval forms occur in the flesh of animals on which these vertebrates feed. The adult tapeworm has no digestive tract but absorbs its nourishment through its body surface. The head or scolex of the worm is provided with means of attachment to the intestinal wall of the host. The remainder of the worm, called the strobila, grows from the scolex and consists of a number, usually large, of segments, or proglottids, identical save in their degree of maturity. Each segment contains male and female reproductive organs, so the entire worm can be thought of as a chain of conjoined hermaphrodites. The segments towards the hind end of the worm are gravid and in effect are bags containing many thousand eggs. Subsequent development of the eggs varies according to the species of worm and will be described in the accounts of the individual parasites.

Unlike the tapeworms, adult trematodes are not confined to the intestine. Those which affect man are found according to the species in the bile ducts, lungs, intestine and blood. Ectopic flukes have been found in many other sites, notably the central nervous system. Most flukes are hermaphrodites, the schistosomes being an exception. They have an intestine which bifurcates and ends blindly at the hind end of the worm. There is no segmentation. The worms are able to attach themselves to the host, usually by means of two suckers, one around the mouth, the other on the ventral surface.

Trematodes have a complex life cycle, differing in detail from one species to another. In general the eggs contain a ciliated larva or miracidium which hatches in water and has a few hours' free life in which to seek out and penetrate the body of a snail. Inside the snail the parasite develops through a succession of stages involving considerable asexual multiplication resulting in the production of large numbers of forms called cercariae which leave the snail and are able directly or indirectly to infect the final host.

114

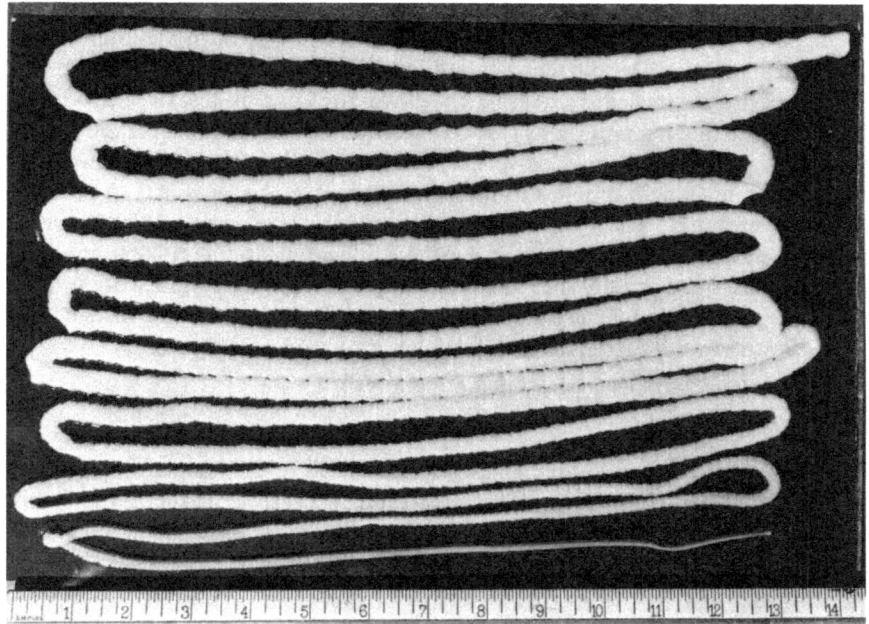

Figure 6.1 *Taenia saginata*, complete worm

THE CESTODES

Taenia saginata

Taenia saginata (Figure 6.1) is the commonest of the tapeworms affecting man, who is the only host of the adult worm. It is worldwide in distribution. The scolex is provided with four sucking discs and is attached to the intestinal wall usually between 40–50 cm beyond the duodenojejunal junction. The rest of the worm, 4–5 metres in length, loops and trails down the intestine. Gravid segments separate at the rate of about six a day. They are motile and can leave the anus independently of any action by the host. For their contained eggs to develop further these must be swallowed by appropriate intermediate hosts. These are usually domestic cattle. Reindeer are also susceptible to the infection, as are various species of antelope. The eggs hatch in the beast's intestine and the liberated embryos or oncospheres penetrate the intestinal wall, enter the bloodstream and are distributed about the body. Those which develop further do so usually in the heart and voluntary muscles of the animal. In these situations cysticerci form, reaching maturity in about 12 weeks, though their growth rate and longevity are very variable. The mature cysticercus is an invaginated bladder about 1 cm in diameter. At the base of the invagination is a layer of germinal cells from which a scolex grows. The cysticerci may live for up to three years and do not appear to affect the health of the animal.

Human infections result from eating meat containing a living cysticercus. Cysticerci are destroyed by heating to above 56 °C or by freezing at −10 °C for ten days, so consumption of raw or inadequately cooked meat is the way in which people acquire this tapeworm. Should a cysticercus be swallowed the scolex evaginates and attaches to the jejunal mucosa. It then starts to produce segments and in 12 weeks will have grown to its full size when gravid segments will start leaving the body of the host. Single infections are the rule but multiple infections are occasionally met with. If not interfered with by medication there seems no reason to suppose that the tapeworm will not live as long as its host. I have known several instances of infections lasting over 20 years.

Clinical features

Taenia saginata very seldom causes physical harm to the host. Complaints of abdominal discomfort, loss of weight and excessive hunger which are sometimes ascribed to the presence of the parasite are in my opinion imaginary and derive from the natural disgust at the thought of the worm. I have observed that young children with this tapeworm are symptomless and thrive normally, being not yet old enough to have learned to worry about their health, The only common tiresome symptom is the discomfort and occasional embarrassment caused by the involuntary extrusion of segments from the anus. Obstruction of the appendix by a proglottid is a rare complication requiring surgical intervention.

Taenia solium

Taenia solium is everywhere much less common than *T. saginata* which it resembles in general outline. The scolex is furnished with a double row of hooks in addition to four suckers. The worm is about 4 metres long and the segments are slenderer, squarer and more translucent than those of *T. saginata*. The eggs are infective to the pig in whose flesh the cysticerci develop. The adult worm develops in man when pork containing a living cysticercus is swallowed. Unfortunately the eggs are also infective to man, so that people may develop cysticercosis either by the chance ingestion of eggs on contaminated food or by autoinfection from an adult worm present in the intestine. This latter accident may be caused by transfer of eggs from anus to mouth on soiled fingers or by the regurgitation of a gravid segment up the intestine so that it behaves as though it had been swallowed. Instances where tapeworm segments have been vomited are well authenticated, so this method of autoinfection is certainly possible.

The question is sometimes raised whether *T. saginata* can cause human cysticercosis. About a dozen instances of varying degrees of dubiety have been reported. Pawlowski and Schultz[1] give references and discuss the problem. They conclude that the question remains open. Certainly it must be a rare accident if it occurs at all.

Taenia solium is no longer found in north-western Europe and North America save as a rare occasional import. It is not uncommon in Mexico and South America and still persists in eastern and southern Europe. The reason for its disappearance from those countries where it was quite common a century ago is no doubt due to the fact that pigs are kept, housed and fed under much more carefully controlled conditions than cattle.

Clinical features

The adult *T. solium* causes trivial intestinal symptoms or none at all. Nevertheless a person harbouring this worm is a danger to himself and to others because of the risk of cysticercosis. The symptoms of cysticercosis depend upon the location of the parasites. These are mostly in the muscles (Figure 6.2) and subcutaneous tissue where they cause no trouble, but all too often they also develop in their brain, where they provoke epilepsy. This is often accompanied by demoralization and a diminution of intellectual and learning capacity.

Cerebral cysticercosis should be considered as a possible explanation for the sudden development of epilepsy in a previously healthy adult. If a patient has cysticerci in his brain he will almost certainly have them elsewhere and may well have noticed them as small subcutaneous lumps feeling like a pea beneath the skin. If these can be found it is a simple matter to cut one out for examination. Radiography of the musculature is useful because cysticerci in the muscles die after about three years. They then become calcified and have a characteristic radiographic appearance.

The treatment of cerebral cysticercosis is symptomatic and consists of giving sufficient doses of phenobarbitone and epanutin to control or minimize the fits. Surgical removal of the cysts is rarely practicable as they are usually scattered widely about the brain.

Hymenolepis nana

This cestode is of negligible medical importance. It is a cosmopolitan parasite of rats and mice. Human infections are by no means uncommon, especially in children in orphanages and similar communities convenient for parasitological investigation. The worm is 3 to 4 cm long. The scolex has four suckers and a single circle of hooklets. The eggs are of characteristic appearance and if ingested by the larvae of certain beetles and fleas will develop into cysticercoids. Should these insects be eaten by a mouse, rat or man the tapeworms will develop in the intestine. Curiously the eggs are also infective to man and if swallowed the liberated oncospheres will enter the intestinal villi and form

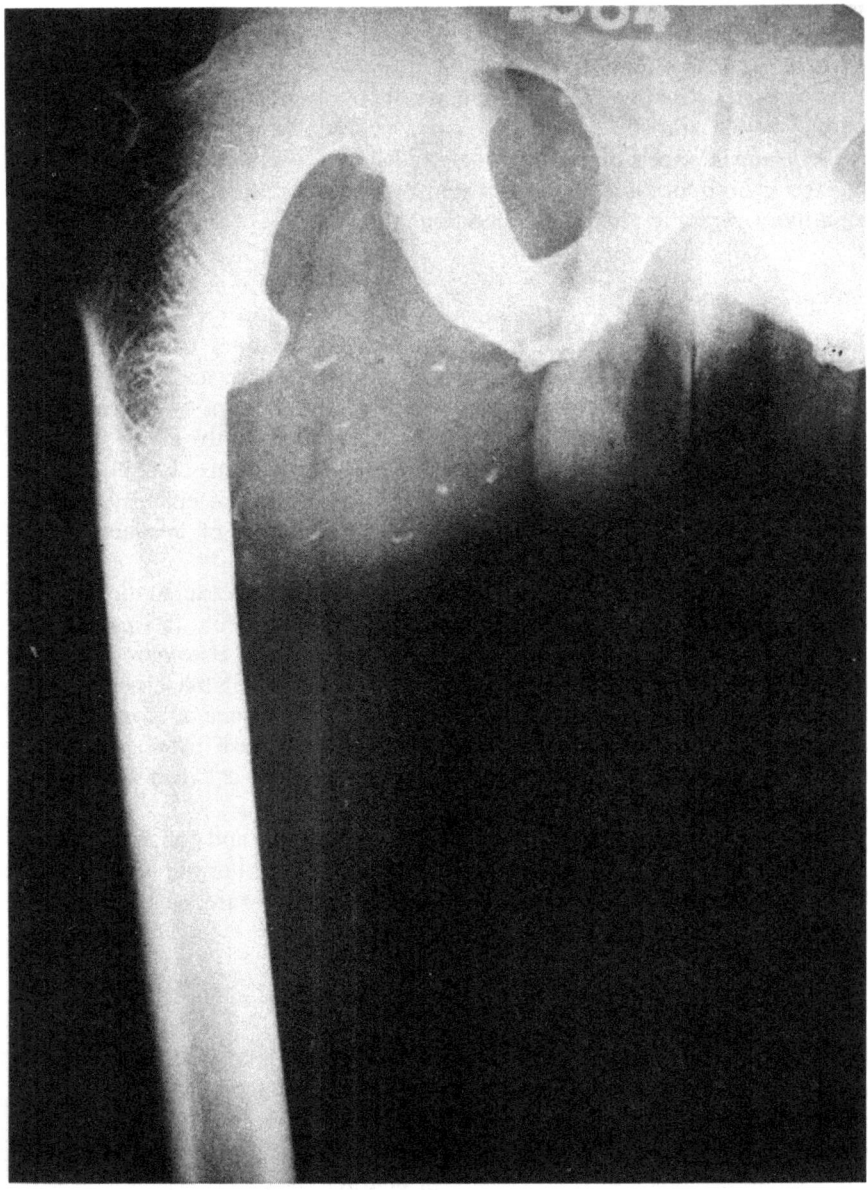

Figure 6.2   *Taenia solium,* calcified cysticerci in thigh muscles

cysticercoids which after an interval of two weeks will emerge into the intestine as adult cestodes. It is probable that some of the eggs produced by these worms will hatch in the intestine and the liberated larvae will penetrate and develop in the villi, thus producing a self-perpetuating infection in man. However, I have yet to see anyone with symptoms attributable to these parasites, whose presence is only recognized by the chance finding of eggs on routine stool examination.

Diphyllobothrium latum

This tapeworm is widely distributed in the north temperate zone and occurs in the intestine of fish-eating mammals. Human infections are nowhere common save in areas where raw or inadequately cooked freshwater fish is an article of diet. In Europe the infection is largely confined to Finland and Scandinavia, and in North America to Alaska and the regions around the Great Lakes. The worm is 5–6 metres in length. The scolex is equipped with two grooves by which it anchors to the intestinal wall. The segments are broader than long and are recognizable by the central ovary shaped like a rosette. Gravid segments (Figure 6.3) and eggs leave the body in the faeces. The eggs are operculate, oval, and 70 μm in length. If they are passed into freshwater, ciliated larvae (coracidia) emerge and swim freely till they perish or are ingested by copepods. They penetrate to the haemocoele of these minute crustaceans and develop into

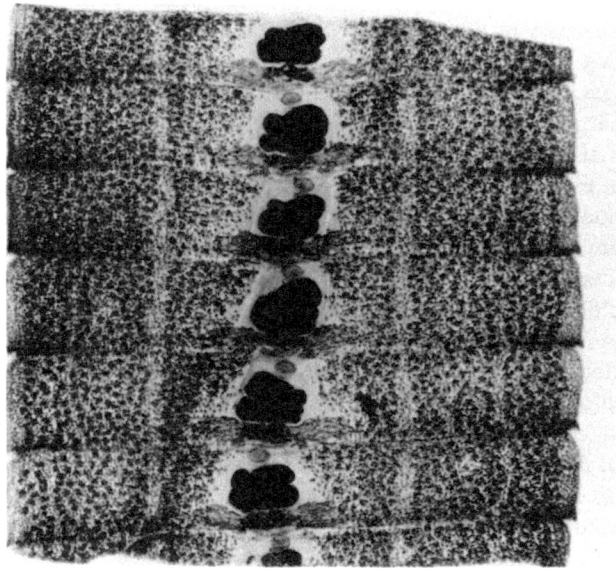

Figure 6.3   *Diphyllobothrium latum*, gravid segments

procercoid larvae. If the infected copepod is swallowed by a fish the procercoid penetrates the fish's intestine and develops in its flesh into a plerocercoid or sparganum. This is a small object on which rudimentary grooves and segmentation can be discerned and is the form infective to man and other animals should it be swallowed. The worm seldom causes symptoms except in Finland where about 3% of infected people develop a megaloblastic anaemia. This is due to a deprivation of vitamin B_{12} which the worm diverts to its own use before it has been absorbed by the host. Removal of the worm cures the anaemia.

Sparganosis

Occasional reports have occurred of human infections with the plerocercoid larva of *Diphyllobothrium* species other than *D. latum*. The methods of infection are to some extent conjectural. These include the swallowing of infected copepods in drinking water, the consumption of flesh of amphibia or reptiles containing spargana and the application of the flesh of such animals to open sores for medicinal purposes. In man the infection becomes manifest when an inflammatory reaction occurs around the sparganum which is recognized only after surgical removal[2].

Echinococcus granulosus

This tapeworm occurs in all the inhabited continents. It is 0.3 to 0.9 cm in length and consists of a scolex and three or four proglottides, the last being gravid (Figure 6.4). The adult worms live in the small intestine of dogs, foxes, wolves and jackals. Eggs are liberated from segments passed in the faeces of these animals and are infective to sheep, cattle, pigs, horses and other herbivores, and also to man. Eggs on infected pastures can remain infective for at least four months. The usual cycle is between sheep and farm dogs. Most human infections are found in those sheep-farming areas where the worms are very prevalent among farm dogs[3]. Probably there are strain differences within the species manifested by the readiness or otherwise with which the eggs can infect the different intermediate host species[4]. Thus in England there is a horse–foxhound cycle and in Poland a pig–dog cycle from which human infections seem not to derive. The parasite is both medically and economically important, medically because it can cause severe and sometimes fatal illness in man and economically because of the substantial monetary loss due to the condemnation of infected offal, estimated as at least £250 000 annually in Britain.

Susceptible intermediate hosts are infected by swallowing the eggs. In herbivores this occurs while grazing on contaminated pastures. Human infections derive from the chance ingestion of eggs on vegetables or by the fondling of an infected dog leading to the transference of eggs from the animal's hair to the mouth by the fingers. This may well be the usual method as many human infec-

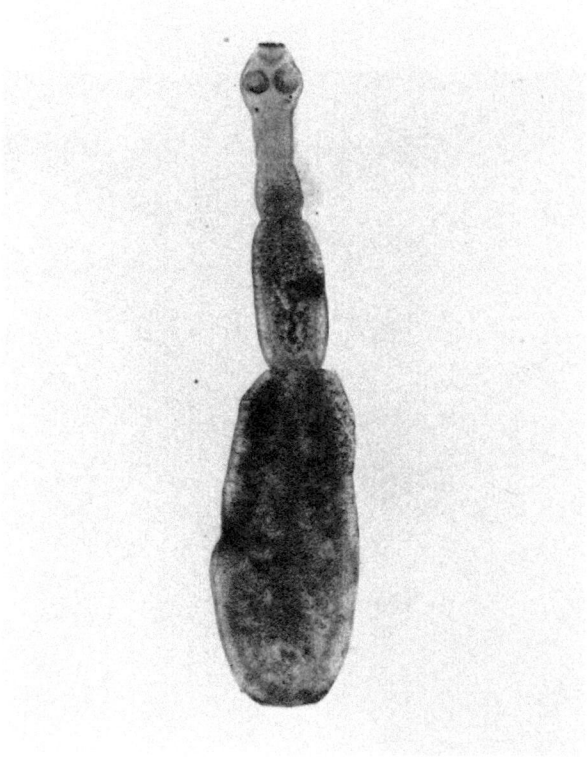

Figure 6.4   *Echinococcus granulosus*, complete worm (Length 0.5 cm)

tions are thought to originate in childhood. Once swallowed, the eggs hatch in the intestine. The liberated oncospheres penetrate the intestinal mucosa and pass along the tributaries of the portal vein to the liver, where for the most part they are filtered out in the portal capillaries and remain. A proportion will pass through the portal circulation and be carried to the lungs where they are held up in the capillaries. A very few may pass this second filter to enter the systemic circulation to be carried to any organ of the body. In human cases the liver and lungs are the affected organs in over 90% of cases and the former organ accounts for almost three-quarters of these. In the affected organ the oncosphere develops into a hydatid cyst (Figure 6.5). The hydatid cyst grows slowly, taking six to twelve months to reach a diameter of about 1 cm. At this stage its characteristic features have become easily demonstrable. These are an outer laminated layer within which is a delicate membrane of germinal cells. These cells form bud-like projections, known as brood capsules, into the fluid-

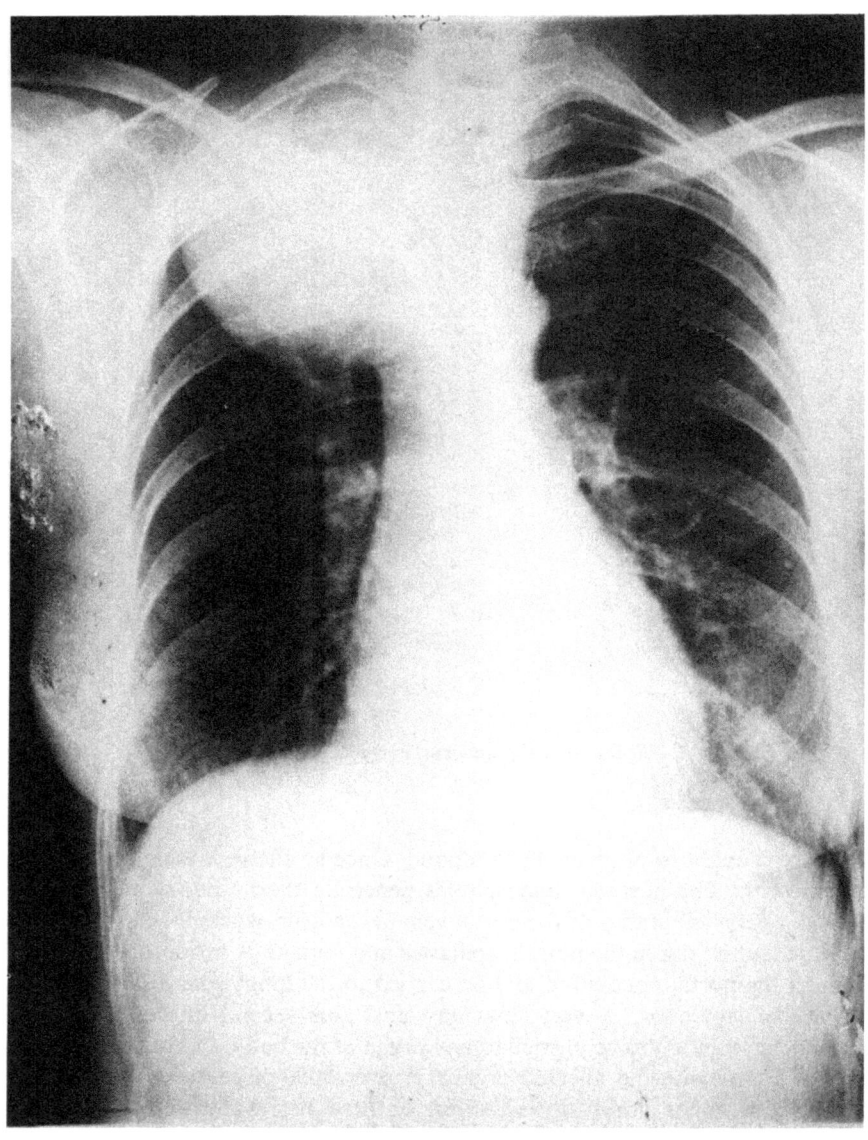

Figure 6.5   Hydatid cyst of lung

filled interior of the cyst. Scoleces are produced within the brood capsules, which as the cyst grows may separate and lie free in the main cyst. Daughter cysts may also form from portions of germinal tissue which have become detached, possibly by trauma. Thus there is great asexual multiplication at this stage, a single hydatid cyst containing many thousands of scoleces, each a potential adult worm (Figure 6.6). Dogs and other definitive hosts acquire the

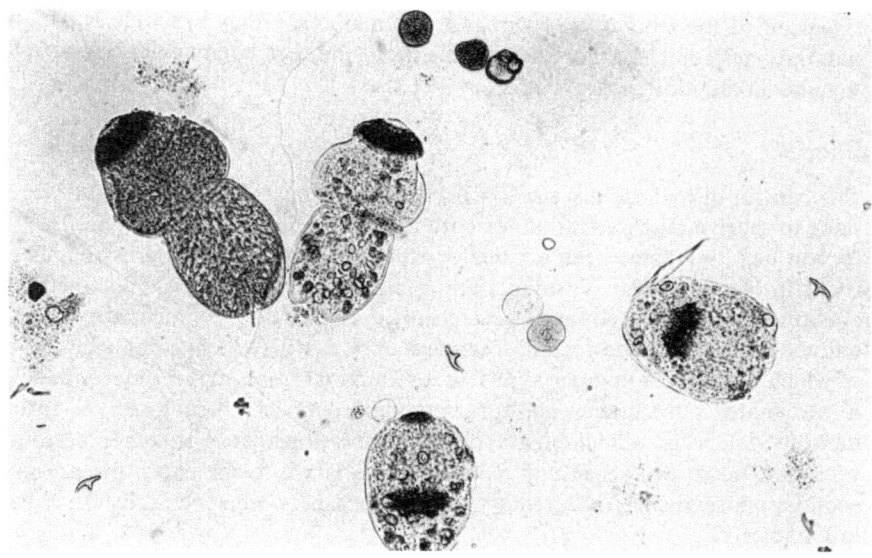

Figure 6.6 *Echinococcus granulosis,* contents of hydatid cyst showing scoleces and hooklets

tapeworms by being fed infected offal, or by scavenging on the carcasses of infected animals which have died on the pastures.

Hydatid cysts in man continue to grow steadily, taking ten or more years to reach a diameter of 15 cm, containing about a litre of fluid in which there is a sediment of daughter cysts, brood capsules and scoleces, the so-called hydatid sand. Hydatid disease in farm animals is usually symptomless, doubtless because they are slaughtered before the cysts have become sufficiently large. However there is some evidence to show that infected sheep thrive less well than healthy animals. In man, too, the infection can be quite symptomless. It is not unusual for a hydatid cyst to die and become calcified without causing the least disturbance to health. Such cases are discovered by chance on radiography. Nevertheless if the cyst continues to enlarge symptoms and signs will sooner or later develop, depending on the situation involved. If the cyst is in the liver or elsewhere in the abdomen it will present as a smooth rounded painless swelling. Pulmonary cysts may cause a localized bulging of the chest wall and are recognizable radiographically. Hydatid cysts may suppurate or rupture. In the latter case there is an immediate danger of anaphylaxis and a remoter one of further cysts developing in adjacent areas from implantation of germinal cells from the primary cyst.

Serological tests are of value in confirming the presence of hydatid disease. The simplest is the Casoni test. The antigen is a filtrate of hydatid fluid. An injection of 0.1 ml is given intradermally and in positive cases a considerable extension of the weal occurs within a few minutes. Other available but more elaborate tests include complement fixation, indirect haemagglutination and enzyme-linked immunosorbent assay (ELISA).

Control

The control of hydatid disease is a matter which has received and should continue to receive much attention for both medical and economic reasons. The infection has long since been eradicated from Iceland. Great progress has been made in New Zealand, Tasmania and more recently in Cyprus. The methods employed are to deny so far as possible the access of dogs to infected carcasses and the registration and regular treatment of dogs with effective antihelminthics of which there are a number available for veterinary use, namely mebendazole, nitroscanate, bunamidine and praziquantel. Any of these given at three-monthly intervals will eliminate *Echinococcus* together with other cestodes such as *Taenia multiceps* and *T. ovis* whose larval forms cause disease and economic loss in sheep. Veterinary control measures are specifically described in Chapter 9.

Echinococcus multilocularis

This cestode resembles *E. granulosus* in its general size and appearance, though there are small anatomical points of difference. The adult worm occurs mainly in foxes and wolves in Northern and Eastern Europe and in North America. It has not been found in Great Britain. Various small rodents, particularly voles, are the usual intermediate hosts. The cysts, which are found in the liver, differ from the hydatid in their proliferative character. The limiting membrane of the cyst does not develop and the germinal layer of cells spreads throughout the affected organ and beyond forming a series of small interconnected or multilocular cysts. Occasional cases of this infection have been reported in man, causing severe or fatal illness as the cysts are hardly susceptible to surgical removal.

The treatment of hydatid disease

Until recently the treatment of hydatid disease has been entirely a matter of surgical judgment and technique. Particular care must be taken at operation to avoid rupturing the cyst with the consequent possibilities of anaphylaxis and the development of secondary cysts from implanted germinal cells. Many surgeons prefer to aspirate a quantity of hydatid fluid from the exposed cyst and to introduce into it a sufficient amount of formalin to give a final concentration of about 10%. This is allowed to act for ten minutes before removal of the cyst is proceeded with, in the hope that the formalin will have killed the germinal cells. What promises to be a considerable advance in the treatment of hydatid disease stems from the work of Heath et al.[5]. This demonstrated the lethal effect of mebendazole on hydatid cysts in artificially infected mice. Subsequently Bekhti et al. reported the successful use of this drug in four human cases of hydatid disease of the liver[6]. The drug was given orally in high doses (400–600 mg three times a day for 21 to 30 days) and in three of the four cases the course had to be repeated once or twice. The end result was the complete regression of the intrahepatic cysts after four to 13 months as demonstrated by ultrasonic echotomography.

Treatment of tapeworm infections

Many substances of uncertain composition and unreliable action have been used in the past to attempt to expel tapeworms from the human intestine. It is only in comparatively recent times that reliable remedies have become available so that what was formerly an exhausting, chancy and even dangerous procedure is now a simple affair of near-certainty. Keeling reviewed the subject and mentioned niclosamide and dichlorophen as the best remedies[7]. Both these drugs kill tapeworms. The older compounds merely caused a temporary disturbance to the parasite allowing it to be swept out of the intestine by a saline purge.

Dichlorophen has the disadvantage that the dose (6 g) is inconveniently large compared with that of niclosamide (2 g). Whichever is used, the tablets should be crushed up in the mouth before swallowing so as to ensure maximum contact between the drug and the scolex of the worm. The treatment is usually given in the morning. There is no need for any interference with the patient's normal activities. Dichlorophen has a slight laxative effect. After treatment the semi-digested remains of the worm are passed during the next day or two. The scolex and anterior segments can seldom be found, so the result of treatment cannot be known with certainty until three or four months have elapsed. If by that time no further segments have left the body, cure can be assumed. The success rate with the large tapeworms is 90% or more. In the case of infections with Hymenolepis it is advisable to repeat the treatment once or twice at three-weekly intervals to deal with worms which have been maturing in the intestinal villi at the time of the first treatment. The propriety of using niclosamide or dichlorophen in T. solium infections is sometimes questioned on the grounds that eggs liberated from the digested segments might cause cysticercosis by autoinfection. The point is a theoretical one which practical experience, particularly in Mexico, has done nothing to confirm. The treatment of children with tapeworms poses no problems. Neither dichlorophen nor niclosamide is significantly absorbed from the intestine so there seems little logic in reducing the dose. Using dichlorophen I found that failures increased sharply at a dose of under 4.5 g. Since niclosamide became available I have given the full dose of 2 g irrespective of the size of the patient. Pregnancy is no contraindication to treatment.

Praziquantel (Droncit) promises to be a useful taenicide. It has been shown to be effective in *D. latum* infections at a dose of 25 mg/kg body weight[8].

THE TREMATODES

Fasciola hepatica

The liver-fluke, *Fasciola hepatica,* is the only trematode of medical interest occurring in the temperate zones. Normally it is parasitic in herbivores, chiefly in sheep. Occasional small human outbreaks are reported from time to time.

The adult fluke (Figure 6.7) is large, measuring about 30 mm in length and 15 mm in breadth. Like most flukes it is flattened dorsoventrally. The flukes are found in the gall-bladder and larger bile ducts. In these sites they lay eggs, each fluke producing some 3000 daily. The eggs are operculated, measuring 130 μm × 70 μm (Figure 6.8). They leave the animal's body in the faeces. In favourable climatic conditions a miracidium (Figure 6.9) develops within nine days, but development may be delayed for several months in adverse circumstances. In water—streams or marshy wet ground—ciliated miracidia will hatch from the eggs to seek the intermediate host. This is a small semiaquatic snail *Limnaea truncatula*. The miracidium enters the soft parts of the snail and makes its way to the digestive gland at the apex of the shell. Here it develops into a sporocyst. This is an amorphous mass of tissue 1 mm long (Figure 6.10). Rediae grow from germinal cells within the sporocyst. Each redia (five or six are formed in each sporocyst) resembles a small fluke 1.5 mm long with a primitive intestine. The rediae leave the sporocyst and their germ cells produce either a second generation of rediae or cercariae. The latter are young flukes equipped with a tail for swimming (Figure 6.11). The development in the snail takes six to seven weeks. A single miracidium may produce over 1000 cercariae. Cercariae will leave the snail's body in wet conditions at temperatures between 10 °C and 26 °C. The cercariae encyst on water-plants and on wet pastures. Their further development awaits their ingestion by a suitable final host. Should this happen the young worms excyst in the intestine, pass through its wall and reach the liver transperitoneally in two or three days. They bore into the liver, wandering and feeding on its substance for five or six weeks before entering the bile ducts and maturing. They start to lay eggs three months after infection.

Liver flukes are of more economic and veterinary than of medical importance. They are the major cause of condemnation of cattle and sheep offal in

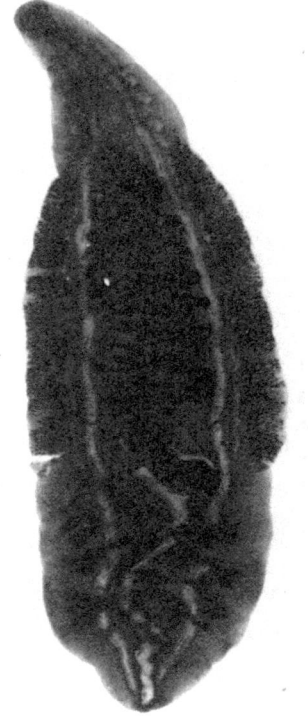

Figure 6.7   *Fasciola hepatica* (Length 2.5 cm × 1.0 cm)

the slaughterhouses, representing an annual loss in Britain of almost £1 million. By contrast human cases of the disease are everywhere unusual. They tend to occur almost exclusively in small outbreaks, often confined to a few families, traceable to the consumption of wild watercress.

Clinical features

The severity of symptoms is, in general, proportional to the weight of the infection, which is light compared with that suffered by sheep and cattle. Typical outbreaks have been described from Algeria[9] and from Britain[10,11]. The symptoms begin from one to three months after infection. Loss of appetite, slight fever, lassitude, and a dull ache in the hepatic region are usual. Urticaria is not uncommon. Examination shows the liver to be tender and sometimes enlarged. A considerable eosinophil leukocytosis is almost always present and it is this finding that suggests a parasitic cause for the illness. Confirmation of the diagnosis should be sought by examination of the faeces for eggs. These cannot

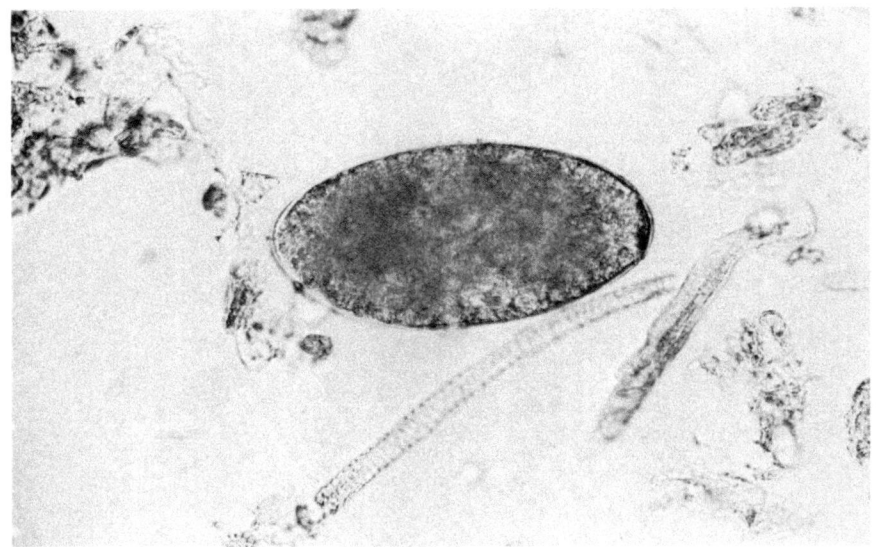

Figure 6.8   *Fasciola hepatica*, egg (Length $130 \times 70 \ \mu$m)

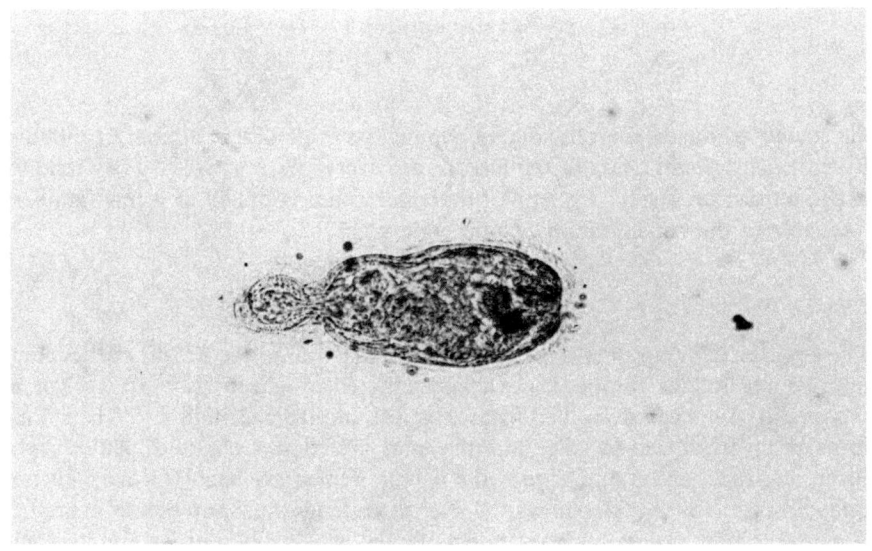

Figure 6.9   Miracidium of *Fasciola hepatica*

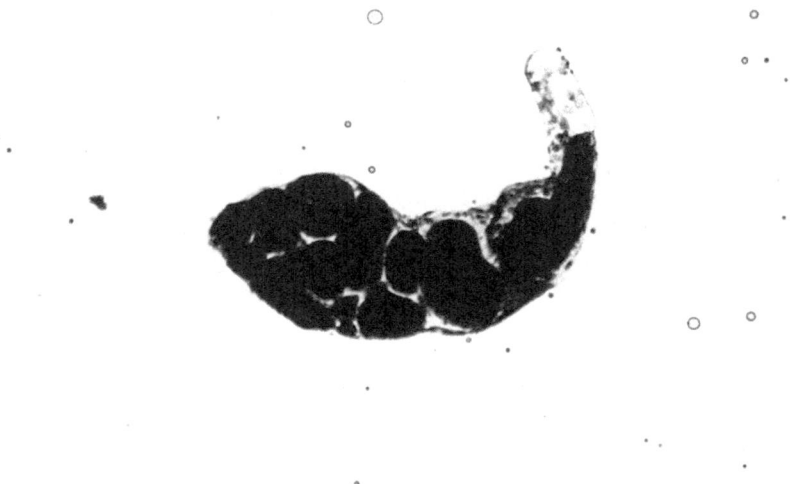

Figure 6.10 Sporocyst of *Fasciola hepatica*, length 4 mm. The interior cell masses develop into rediae

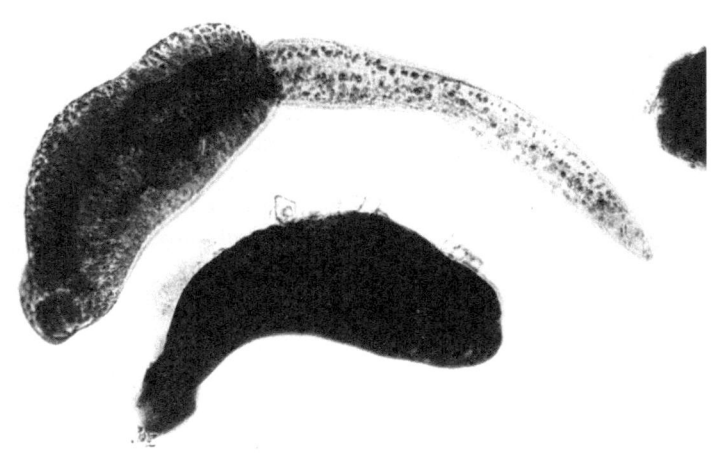

Figure 6.11 Cercaria of *Fasciola hepatica* (Length 1 mm)

always be found, either because the flukes have failed to mature, or because sufficient time for their maturation has not yet elapsed. In such cases serological tests provide confirmatory evidence.

Treatment

Emetine and dehydroemetine have both been used successfully for treating human facioliasis, the dose being 1 mg/kg body weight given subcutaneously daily for 10 days. Both drugs may harm the myocardium, so it is necessary for the patient to be at rest during the course and afterwards to return gradually to full activity. Bithional has also been effective, but is not easily obtained. It is given orally, 4 mg/kg body weight, in divided doses on alternate days for 10 treatment days. It usually causes nausea and vomiting. More effective drugs are available for veterinary use, namely rafoxamide and oxyclozanide, and there seems no reason to suppose that they would not be equally useful in human infections.

Exotic trematode infection—Schistosomes

With the exception of a small focus of *Schistosoma haematobium* in Portugal the schistosomes of man are not found in the Western world save as imported cases, though these are not uncommon. Adult schistosomes live in the veins around the urinary bladder (*S. haematobium*) and large intestine (*S. mansoni* and *S. japonicum*). The worms are of separate sexes. The female lays eggs, some of which make their way through the wall and into the cavity of the adjacent viscus, so leaving the body in the urine or faeces. Other eggs stick in the wall of the viscus, and others drift away in the venous return to be filtered out either in the lungs (*S. haematobium*) or liver (*S. mansoni* and *S. japonicum*). Those eggs leaving the body will hatch if passed into fresh water. The emerging miracidia are infective to various species of aquatic snail in which they undergo asexual reproduction resulting in the production of large numbers of cercariae which are shed into the water. Human infections derive from bathing or wading in infected water. The cercariae penetrate the skin, enter the circulation, mature in the portal venules in the liver and having matured pass down the mesenteric veins to their site of election.

Clinical features

Passage of cercariae through the skin is sometimes followed by an itching eruption at the site. This phenomenon, 'bather's itch' is also caused by the schistosomes of aquatic birds whose cercariae are able to penetrate human skin but cannot complete their development in man. In such cases the dermatitis is more severe and prolonged than in natural infections. Cercarial dermatitis due to bird schistosomes has a deleterious effect on the amenity value of some

North American lakes. Maturation of the schistosomes in the liver may produce a period of irregular fever, urticaria, liver tenderness and eosinophilia, starting about one month after infection and lasting for two or three weeks. This is present regularly in *S. japonicum* infection, where it has been given the name of Katayama disease, but is also seen in *S. mansoni* and less often in *S. haematobium* infection. When the schistosomes have started to lay eggs the symptoms are referable to the bladder (*S. haematobium*) or to the intestine and liver (*S. mansoni* and *S. japonicum*). Intermittent painless haematuria is almost always the presenting symptom in *S. haematobium* infection. Infections with *S. mansoni* in visitors to endemic areas are as a rule light and symptomless. They come to light on routine screening of travellers on their return from abroad by finding ova in the faeces. There is usually an associated eosinophilia of moderate degree and serological tests for schistosomiasis are positive, though these do not distinguish between the different species of schistosome and are of secondary importance compared with the finding of eggs. In late cases of *S. mansoni* and *S. japonicum* infections there is more or less liver damage due to periportal fibrosis around the eggs which have been held up in the portal capillaries. This can lead to portal hypertension, splenomegaly, ascites and oesophageal varices, but these complications are seldom seen except in natives of the endemic areas, who have had heavy infections for long periods.

Treatment

S. haematobium infections are the easiest to cure and *S. japonicum* the hardest. Several drugs are available. The antimony compound stibocaptate (Astiban) is effective in all three forms of schistosomiasis. It is given as an intramuscular injection of a freshly made 10% solution. The dose is 6 mg/kg body weight given on alternate days on five occasions. Niridazole (Ambilhar) has the advantage of oral administration. A dose of 8 mg/kg body weight three times a day for five days is sufficient to cure *S. haematobium* infections. A longer course is required for the other forms. Hycanthone (Etrenol) is very suitable for treating the light infections with *S. haematobium* and *S. mansoni* seen in persons returned from the endemic zones. A single intramuscular injection of 3 mg/kg is all that is needed in such cases. Treated cases should be re-examined after an interval of not less than three months, when if no living eggs can be found cure can be assumed.

References

1. Pawlowski, Z. and Schultz, M. J. (1972). Taeniasis and cysticercosis (*Taenia saginata*). *Adv. Parasitol.*, **10**, 269
2. Markell, E. K. and Huber, S. L. (1964). A case of human sparganosis. *Am. J. Med.*, **37**, 491
3. Walters, T. M. H. (1977). Hydatid disease in Wales. *Trans. R. Soc. Trop. Med. Hyg.*, **71**, 105

4. Smyth, J. D. (1977). Strain differences in *Echinococcus granulosus*, with special reference to the status of equine hydatidosis in the United Kingdom. *Trans. R. Soc. Trop. Med. Hyg.*, **71**, 93

5. Heath, D. D., Christie, M. J. and Chevis, R. A. F. (1975). The lethal effect of mebendazole on secondary *Echinococcus granulosus*, cysticerci of *Taenia pisiformis* and tetrathrydia of *Metacestoides cerci. Parasitology*, **70**, 273

6. Bekhti, A., Schaaps, J. P., Capron, M., Dessaint, J. P., Santore, F., and Capron, A. (1977). Treatment of hepatic hydatid disease with mebendazole: preliminary results in four cases. *Br. Med. J.*, **2**, 1047

7. Keeling, J. E. (1968). The chemotherapy of cestode infections. *Adv. Chemother.*, **3**, 109

8. Bylund, G., Bong, B. and Wikgren, K. (1977). Tests with a new compound (praziquantel) against *Diphyllobothrium latum. J. Helminth.*, **51**, 115

9. Combaras, A. (1966). La distomatose hepatique en Algerie. *Ann. Parasit. Hum. Comp.*, **41**, 71

10. Ashton, W. L. G., Boardman, F. L., D'Sa, C. J., Everall, P. H., and Houghton, A. W. J. (1970). Human fascioliasis in Shropshire. *Br. Med. J.*, **3**, 500

11. Hardman, E. W., Jones, R. L. H. and Davies, A. H. (1970). Fascioliasis, a large outbreak. *Br. Med. J.*, **3**, 502

7
Protozoa

H. M. GILLES

GENERAL DESCRIPTION

Protozoa are unicellular animals. The single cell which carries out all the functions comprises a cytoplasm which contains one or more nuclei. The nucleus consists of a membrane with a network of fine filaments inside it; on this membrane and on the enclosed network are arranged granules of chromatin. Inside the nucleus is a mass, usually central in position and roughly circular in shape, known as the karyosome.

Protozoa feed by engulfing food in solid form in the interior of 'food vacuoles' in the cytoplasm or absorbing it in liquid state. Protozoa are variably motile. The movement is carried out by means of pseudopodia (temporary cytoplasmic processes), flagella (permanent organelles) or cilia. Certain parasites which are active at one stage may be motionless at another when they enclose themselves in a resistant tough membrane wall, known as a cyst. The methods of reproduction among the protozoa are very diverse, e.g. by binary fission, asexual or sexual multiplication A (Table 7.1).

Virtually all the pathogenic protozoa can now be found in developed countries but the ones that occur with any degree of frequency are *Entamoeba histolytica, Toxoplasma gondii, Giardia lamblia,* and the most important of all, the Plasmodia, i.e. *P. falciparum* and *P. vivax* in particular. The other protozoan genera, i.e. *Trypanosoma; Leishmania; Naegleria; Isospora; Balantidium; Trichinomas;* and *Babesia* are mainly confined to developing countries and are only occasionally encountered in medical practice in Europe, North America and Australasia.

ENTAMOEBA HISTOLYTICA

This species occurs in man and is pathogenic. The parasite lives in the large intestine causing ulceration of the mucosa with consequent diarrhoea. Secondary

Table 7.1   Classification of Phylum Protozoa†

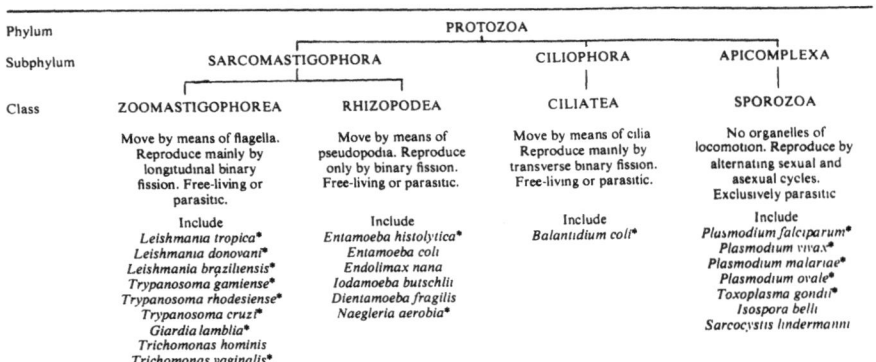

Phylum	PROTOZOA			
Subphylum	SARCOMASTIGOPHORA		CILIOPHORA	APICOMPLEXA
Class	ZOOMASTIGOPHOREA	RHIZOPODEA	CILIATEA	SPOROZOA
	Move by means of flagella. Reproduce mainly by longitudinal binary fission. Free-living or parasitic.	Move by means of pseudopodia. Reproduce only by binary fission. Free-living or parasitic.	Move by means of cilia. Reproduce mainly by transverse binary fission. Free-living or parasitic.	No organelles of locomotion. Reproduce by alternating sexual and asexual cycles. Exclusively parasitic
	Include	Include	Include	Include
	Leishmania tropica*	Entamoeba histolytica*	Balantidium coli*	Plasmodium falciparum*
	Leishmania donovani*	Entamoeba coli		Plasmodium vivax*
	Leishmania braziliensis*	Endolimax nana		Plasmodium malariae*
	Trypanosoma gamiense*	Iodamoeba butschlii		Plasmodium ovale*
	Trypanosoma rhodesiense*	Dientamoeba fragilis		Toxoplasma gondii*
	Trypanosoma cruzi*	Naegleria aerobia*		Isospora belli
	Giardia lamblia*			Sarcocystis lindermanni
	Trichomonas hominis			
	Trichomonas vaginalis*			

*   Serious pathogens
†   This classification is now in a state of flux with the advent of biochemical taxonomy.

lesions may occur, most commonly in the liver but other tissues can be affected, e.g. lungs, brain, genital organs, and skin[1,2].

Geographical distribution

Amoebiasis has a worldwide distribution but clinical disease occurs most frequently in tropical and subtropical latitudes. An international conference on amoebiasis was held in Mexico City in 1975 and the proceedings have been published[3]. In Great Britain, 255 cases of *E. histolytica* were reported in 1976 while in 1975, 2775 occurred in the United States.

Morphology

The amoebic trophozoites (unencysted amoeba) consists of a small mass of cytoplasm capable of amoeboid movement, its size is generally between 10 μm and 40 μm. The cytoplasm shows differentiation into an outer layer of ectoplasm which is clear and translucent, and an inner mass of endoplasm which is rather dense. Within the endoplasm there is a spherical nucleus, bounded by a thin limiting membrane on which small granules of chromatin are arranged in a regular pattern of dots. Inside the nucleus is a slightly larger granule called the karyosome. The nucleus is not readily visible in fresh preparations, unless the amoeba is moving fairly actively. Forms which are dividing may show two nuclei. In the endoplasm are found also vacuoles with contents such as particles of food material, portions of leukocytes and occasionally bacteria.

The cysts are round or oval in outline, refractile, somewhat pearly in colour, with a definite cyst wall; cysts containing one, two or four nuclei may be present in the same sample of faeces. They measure about 12 μm in diameter, ranging between 10 μm and 15 μm. Since the cysts are much smaller than the tissue-invading unencysted forms, they might be derived from them by contraction; more probably, however, the parasites develop into special small precystic forms which then become enclosed in a cyst wall.

The newly-formed cyst, like the amoeba from which it arises, has one nucleus; it also contains a glycogen mass, and, usually, characteristic refractile rod-like structures with rounded ends, called chromidial bars or chromatoid bodies. Most frequently there are two chromidial bars, though there may be one or many, and they may extend almost across the diameter of the cyst, or be shorter. As the cyst grows older, two changes occur in it, affecting the nucleus and the glycogen mass. The single nucleus divides into two, and each of these divides again into two, giving rise to the four-nucleated cyst, which is the typical fully developed cyst, and the glycogen mass and chromidial bars are used up gradually and disappear. In fresh unstained films of faeces containing *Entamoeba histolytica* cysts, the nuclei of the cyst are difficult to see and the glycogen mass is seldom visible, but the chromatoid bodies, if present, are prominent as stout refractile rods, which can be seen fairly easily if the proper degree of light is used and the cyst contents are carefully focused. In iodine-stained specimens of faeces, the cysts are yellow to light brown, and the nuclei are clearly seen; the glycogen mass appears light brown with the centre more deeply stained, the colour fading away gradually at the edge into the surrounding cytoplasm; the chromatoid bodies are not stained by the iodine and cannot usually be seen.

Life cycle

The amoeba multiplies by binary fission. It lives in the lumen of the large intestine where under suitable conditions it invades the mucous membrane and submucosa. If red blood cells are available, the amoeba will ingest them. When diarrhoea occurs, amoebae are expelled to the exterior as such, and then are found in the freshly passed fluid stools. Amoebae are very sensitive to environmental changes, and so are short-lived outside the body. When there is no diarrhoea and other conditions are favourable for encystation, the amoebae cease feeding, become spherical, secrete a cyst wall and the nucleus divides twice to form the characteristic mature four-nucleate cyst.

The cyst is the infective form, and when ingested hatches in the lower part of the small intestine or upper part of the large intestine and a four-nucleate amoeba emerges from the cyst. After a series of nuclear and cytoplasmic divisions, each multinucleate amoeba gives rise to eight uninucleate amoebae, which establish themselves and multiply in the large intestine.

The sizes of the cysts produced by individual strains vary from 7μm to 15μm in diameter; they can be divided into two groups, those strains producing cysts over 10μm and those below 10μm in diameter. The strains producing small cysts are now held to belong to a separate species, *E. hartmanni*. Infections with *E. hartmanni* are symptomless.

Experimental infection of rats and kittens has proved useful for assessing the virulence of various strains of *E. histolytica*. But in spite of much effort, the basis for pathogenicity has not been unequivocally determined.

In order to establish itself in the intestine *E. histolytica* requires an association with bacteria but it is still not clear how the amoebae invade the intestinal mucosa. *In vitro* cultivation has been achieved in a variety of media in the presence of bacteria, and it has been demonstrated that trophozoites possess proteolytic enzymes capable of digesting the epithelium of the large intestine. Thus, gelatinases, hyaluronidase activity and other proteolytic enzymes have been demonstrated in strains of *E. histolytica*, but the presence of these substances has not specifically been correlated with the pathogenicity of a strain[4]. The mechanism of host tissue destruction has been clarified by studies of the ultrastructure of the rectal tissue from dysentery patients[5], and the caecal mucosa of infected guinea pigs[6,7]. Diamond and Mattern[8] have reviewed the work on the virus of *E. histolytica* but the relevance of these viruses to virulence is uncertain. Within the true *E. histolytica* group of amoebae some differences have been found in DNA base composition and genome size as well as by immunofluorescence. The ultrastructure of trophozoites has been described by Henley *et al.*[9] using a freeze-etching technique.

E. histolytica infection may extend directly from the large intestine to surrounding structures within the abdomen, or it may be spread by artificial and natural orifices to the surrounding skin. More commonly the infection spreads extra-intestinally by blood-born embolism, especially to the liver by the portal circulation; from here it can extend directly to neighbouring structures, e.g. pleura and lung or the pericardium. Alternatively embolic spread may occur to the brain or other organs.

Mode of transmission

In most populations where *E. histolytica* is endemic, prevalence remains stable and the incidence and morbidity rates are low. Individual infections are often of long duration and liable to spontaneous loss; reinfection is common. These features of amoebic infection, especially measurement of the low transmission rates, create problems for the epidemiologist[10]. The disease is spread by cyst passers, who may be divided into two main groups: (a) convalescents who have recovered from an acute attack, and (b) individuals who can recall no clinical evidence of infection. The latter possibly are the more common source of infection, even in countries with high standards of hygiene. Bad sanitation is more important than climate in the predominance of overt infection in the tropics. Carrier rates of *E. histolytica* among symptomless subjects have varied between 20% and 80% in some communities. The parasite can be transmitted by direct contact through the contaminated hands of cyst carriers, e.g. in institutions; it is also transmitted indirectly by means of contaminated food, such as raw vegetables fertilized with fresh human faeces, and through the intermediary of food handlers and flies. Infected water has occasionally been held responsible for the transmission of large outbreaks of the disease.

Although several animals harbour *E. histolytica*—monkeys, dogs, pigs, rats, cats—they are thought to be of no epidemiological importance in human infections. Amoebiasis is not infrequently a house or family infection.

Among factors influencing the epidemiology of the disease we have to consider age, sex, race, the effect of immunity, the role of the concomitant infection, and the influence of diet[11-13].

Pathology

The large intestine is usually the primary site of amoebic infection and in order of frequency, the regions affected are the caecum, flexures, descending colon, and rectum. The appendix is sometimes involved and rarely the ileum may be invaded.

Macroscopically the large intestine may be studded with discrete ulcers with pointing overhanging edges, the intervening mucosa being relatively normal. These 'vertical' deep ulcers are in contrast to the superficial shallow, spreading ulcers seen in bacillary dysentery. At necropsy, however, the lesions are usually much more extensive. The ulcers spread laterally in the submucosa and become confluent. Large areas of mucosa are lost and greenish shaggy sloughs may involve the muscle coat and extend even to the serosa. In other cases a stringy, seaweed-like slough may cover most of the mucosa leaving only occasional islands of recognizable tissue. In patients whose host/parasite balance has been altered either by drugs, concurrent disease or pregnancy, the whole of the mucosa may be sloughing, dark, and gangrenous and the underlying amoebic infection may be difficult to detect. The wall of the bowel is thickened and friable[14,15].

Penetration of the basement membrane and muscularis is usual in lesions seen at necropsy. The amoebae spread laterally beneath the muscularis and intestinal epithelium, forming large 'flask-shaped' or 'water-bottle' ulcers. These ulcers have overhanging edges and consist of a flask-shaped zone of necrosis surrounded by a low-grade inflammatory reaction with lymphocytes and macrophages predominant. A variable fibroblastic reaction is present. Amoebae are present at the periphery of the lesion in the submucosa and muscle layers. They may also be seen in the necrotic tissue itself. They are present singly or in small groups and are round or oval bodies slightly larger than the macrophages and have a clear zone surrounding them. They stain positively by a periodic acid Schiff technique. The presence of secondary bacterial infection determines the presence or absence of acute inflammatory cells. The gross and macroscopic pathology of the liver during amoebic dysentery has been described by Ramachandran *et al*.[16].

Liver abscess (Figure 7.1) is the most common extra-intestinal complication of intestinal amoebiasis. The abscess is usually single but multiple abscesses are

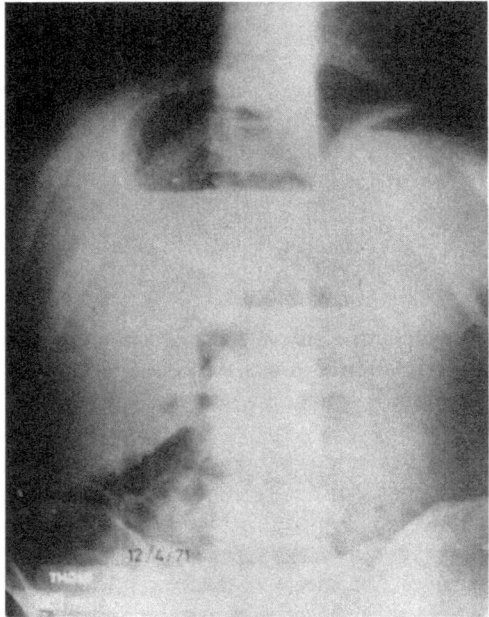

Figure 7.1   X-ray of amoebic liver abscess

not uncommon. The right lobe of the liver is most frequently affected, especially the posterior portion of the dome. The left lobe may, however, be solely involved. Bile would appear to destroy the amoebae as the gall bladder is never affected. In over 50% of patients with amoebic infections of the liver there may be no evidence of amoebic infection on stool examination. The amoebae cause lysis of the parenchymal cells of the liver primarily in the periportal region. An extending necrosis follows and the abscess cavity may reach a diameter of 12 cm. The cavity contains sterile, chocolate-coloured fluid, the result of the lysis of liver cells, granular debris, and few inflammatory cells. Amoebae may or may not be present in the pus. Histologically the wall of the abscess consists of necrotic tissue and compressed liver parenchyma containing a variable infiltrate of monocytes, plasma cells, lymphocytes, and fibroblasts. Amoebae may be seen in the area of coagulative necrosis or in the least affected compressed liver tissue.

Clinical features

Clinical manifestations of amoebiasis include amoebic dysentery with or without complications, and amoeboma which is a localized form involving the gut walls and sometimes confused clinically with neoplasm[17]. Extra-intestinal amoebic infection leads most commonly to liver abscess.

Asymptomatic intestinal infections are the rule in those acquiring their infections in temperate climates.

The symptoms of amoebic dysentery may appear within a week or two of infection or be delayed for months or years. The onset is usually gradual, with some looseness for a few days followed by evacuation of up to six or eight, but rarely more than a dozen, mucoid blood-stained motions a day. Colic and tenesmus are unusual unless there is a lesion immediately inside the anus. On physical examination there may be no signs of significance. Occasionally, and especially during more acute attacks, there is palpable thickening, with tenderness on pressure, of the caecum or of the descending colon and sigmoid flexure. There is no fever of significance and little prostration. The duration of an attack of amoebic dysentery of ordinary severity may be a few days or it may last for some weeks; it then usually subsides spontaneously. There follows a period of remission which may last days, weeks, months, or even years; during this the patient not uncommonly is constipated. Another attack of dysentery then follows. This sequence of attacks of dysentery followed by intermissions associated with constipation, which may continue for years and even for the duration of the patient's life, constitutes the classical picture of amoebic dysentery. At any time complications, especially an amoebic liver abscess, may develop; they do so in about one-fifth of neglected cases.

In some cases, for instance in patients who are undernourished or are suffering from other debilitating diseases, attacks may be prolonged and may be very severe, sometimes fatal.

Amoebic dysentery is sometimes very acute and fulminating, with sudden onset, swinging fever, chills, sweating and very severe dysentery, dehydration and prostration. In such cases the stools are liquid, with flecks of faecal matter and variable amounts of blood and mucus. There may be severe intestinal haemorrhages or perforation, followed by amoebic peritonitis. The mortality in untreated cases is high. Attacks of this kind have frequently been reported in South Africa, usually in Bantu.

The direct complications of an intestinal infection are haemorrhage, often considerable, from erosion of a large vessel in the bowel wall; extension of the infection through the bowel wall, with the formation of amoebic granulomata (amoebomata); and frank sudden perforation. In addition to sudden perforation of an amoebic ulcer, with development of an acute surgical abdomen, a form of slow leakage through an extensively diseased bowel may result in peritonitis. The latter occurs only in the severe fulminating type of amoebic dysentery. All complications are rare in the classical case of average severity.

The clinical picture of amoebic liver abscess develops most frequently during an intermission in chronic amoebic dysentery or colitis. The patient usually gives a history of dysentery or intermittent loose diarrhoea, but there may be no such previous evidence of infection. Only rarely does the picture develop during an attack of dysentery or active colitis, although liver enlargement and tenderness may occur during the attack.

There is usually only one large abscess, but occasionally there are two or more and sometimes many small lesions. The volume of the contents of the lesion may be as much as 500–1500 ml.

In the early stages the patient complains of discomfort and fullness in the liver region. The liver enlarges and becomes tender, the tenderness becoming intensified over the area of the abscess. Moderate fever develops which may at first be intermittent but becomes remittent. Sweating is severe, especially at night. The patient is very anorexic and beings to lose weight. For a time he feels better than his clinical state warrants, but he becomes progressively more toxic and eventually prostrated.

By the time the abscess has formed, there is high swinging or intermittent fever, with drenching night sweats. The patient complains of intense discomfort and tenderness over the liver, particularly over the region occupied by the abscess. The liver is often enlarged and tender, sometimes bulging in the abscess area, where the tenderness is intense and very localized. The maximum tenderness is commonly on the right intercostally in the lateral or medial–lateral lines over the lower rib cage. The chest wall and abdomen are sometimes obviously bulging in this area[18].

Movement of the affected side of the chest is greatly restricted. The patient finds deep breathing painful and the respiration rate is consequently increased. On whichever side of the liver the abscess has developed, the hepatic dullness is increased upwards; when the lesion is in the right lobe, the shadow is increased upward and X-ray will reveal that the diaphragm is pushed up and is usually immobile. The liver edge is usually palpable well away from the abscess area and may project two or three fingers-breadth below the costal margin; it is firm and tender.

Jaundice although uncommon does occur. Most cases have a moderate degree of leukocytosis, ranging from 12 000 to 15 000 cells per mm³, most of which are polymorphs. The ESR is raised.

There may be signs of pulmonary involvement, usually above the raised immobile diaphragm at the base of the right lung in which there may be some atelectasis; pleural effusion is not uncommon in the same region. When the hepatic lesion has broken through the diaphragm into the lung, the abscess contents may reach the bronchi and the patient develops a cough and may discharge the classical 'anchovy sauce' sputum which usually contains amoebae and lysed liver material.

If the progress of the abscess is not arrested by specific treatment, it will erode into adjacent structures, that is, through the diaphragm into the thoracic cavity or into the pericardial sac (especially when the abscess is in the left lobe of the liver), through the peritoneum into the peritoneal cavity, through the chest or abdominal wall to the exterior or into contiguous organs or tissues within the abdomen.

Embolic spread may result in abscess formation in other organs, sometimes in the brain, with localizing signs depending on the area in which the lesion develops. It is probable that most exotic lesions of this sort are derived from an initial amoebic abscess in the liver, but primary brain and lung lesions have been reported; in the latter case the pus coughed up in the sputum is creamy white and not anchovy.

Diagnosis

The clinical diagnosis of amoebiasis has to be confirmed by identification of *E. histolytica*. During an attack of amoebic dysentery the motions are loose, offensive, and contain mucus and blood; faecal elements are always present. On microscopical examination motile amoebae, some with engorged red cells, will be found in the freshly passed stool or in specimens removed at sigmoidoscopy or proctoscopy.

In asymptomatic infections, and during remission, the stool is semiformed and contains *E. histolytica* cysts. They can be seen to contain one or more barshaped chromatoid bodies and staining with iodine reveals one to four nuclei and a glycogen mass. Repeated stool examinations (six to ten) should be made before absence of infection can confidently be assumed. Concentration techniques for cysts are available, and cultural methods may assist diagnosis in scanty infections.

Amoebic ulceration is commonly found in the rectum and sigmoid, so that sigmoidoscopic examination often affords valuable information. Usually, small yellow ulcers with surrounding hyperaemia are seen, while in between the ulcers the mucous membrane is not inflamed. In chronic cases, amoebic lesions may appear as 'pin-point craters' irregularly disposed (Figure 7.2).

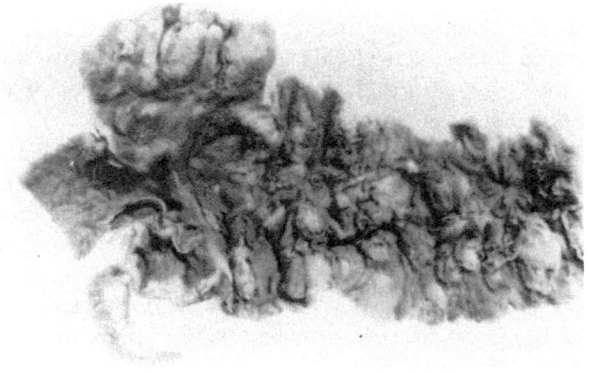

Figure 7.2   Ulcers in the caecum in fulminating amoebic dysentery following steroid therapy

The diagnosis of extra-intestinal amoebiasis can be difficult and atypical clinical presentations especially of amoebic liver abscess are not uncommon[19]. Concomitant amoebic dysentery may be present in 5–10% of patients. *E. histolytica* frequently are not found in the stools, and a polymorphonuclear leukocytosis may not be present. Diagnostic aspiration may produce the typical 'chocolate coloured' or 'anchovy sauce' pus and immediate direct examination of the abscess contents may reveal amoebae.

Liver abscess may cause a raised right diaphragm which shows restricted movement. Though the normal shape of the right dome may be preserved, localized bulging or 'humping' is sometimes seen. A small pleural effusion is frequently recorded while basal atelectasis usually linear in appearance also occurs[20]. Diagnostic methods other than simple radiography that have been used include aspiration with air or lipiodol replacement, splenic cenography, and the induction of a pneumoperitoneum. Isotope scanning of the liver and ultrasonic sounding have also been used for defining liver abscesses. Amoebic lung abscesses are usually thick-walled and occur mainly in the anterior basal segment of the right lower lobe; consolidation with or without abscess formation may also occur.

The relative merits of three diagnostic tests and the cellulose membrane precipitin test have been reviewed by Stamm *et al.*[21,22]. The indirect fluorescent antibody test is a good clinical screening test, while the gel diffusion precipitin test also shows a close correlation with clinical disease. The most promising new serological developments are countercurrent immunoelectrophoresis and the enzyme-linked immunosorbent test[23–25]. Isotope scans, hepatic arteriography and ultrasound are all useful ancillary diagnostic techniques [26–28].

Treatment

Metronidazole (Flagyl) continues to give good results in both amoebic dysentery and liver abscess. Parenteral metronidazole is now available[29]. Tinidazole has also given good results[30].

Asymptomatic intestinal amoebiasis can be treated by either diloxanide furoate, 500 mg orally thrice daily for 10 days, or di-iodohydroxyquinoline (Diodoquin) 600 mg thrice daily for 21 days.

Attacks of acute amoebic dysentery can be treated by metronidazole 800 mg orally thrice daily for 5 days. As an alternative emetine hydrochloride may be used in a dosage of 1 mg per kg body weight (not exceeding 65 mg in any one day) intramuscularly or subcutaneously as a single dose or in two divided doses, each day for 4–10 days.

Dehydroemetine may be given as an alternative to emetine, in doses of 1.5 mg per kg body weight (not exceeding 90 mg in any one day).

Neither of these drugs should be given to patients with cardiac disease; they are best avoided in pregnancy and in aged patients. They should be given only when the patient is in bed and under supervision.

The emetine injections are stopped once the acute signs have ceased and treatment of the intestinal infection is continued with tetracycline and diloxanide furoate or Diodoquin.

For amoebic abscess of the liver metronidazole 800 mg thrice daily for 5 days is usually adequate. This regimen will also clear any contiguous complication or intestinal infection that may be present. It may be combined with chloroquine.

Alternatively, a combined course may be given, consisting of emetine hydrochloride 65 mg or dehydroemetine 90 mg intramuscularly as a single dose or in two divided doses daily for 4–12 days depending on the clinical response. Chloroquine 600 mg (base) is given immediately, followed by 300 mg (base) in 6 hours then 150 mg (base) twice daily for up to 28 days. The possible gut infection is controlled by diloxanide furoate, 500 mg thrice daily for 10 days.

Aspiration is needed if chemotherapy does not bring relief or if there is a mass with very localized tenderness, or if the abscess appears to be pointing in a particular spot. Big abscesses need aspiration and are indicated by a grossly elevated and immobilized hemidiaphragm (usually right).

Control measures including food hygiene which are effective against enteric bacterial infections will usually prove effective for amoebiasis.

TOXOPLASMA GONDII

This is a coccidian parasite which inhabits the viscera, musculature, lymphatic glands and the central nervous system of man as well as of a large variety of animals and birds.

Geographical distribution

The parasite has a worldwide distribution. In 1976, 611 cases were reported in Great Britain.

Morphology

The individual parasites are crescent-shaped, measuring 4–6 μm in length by 2 to 3 μm in breadth. One end of the parasite is pointed, the other is bluntly pointed or rounded and is broader. The nucleus is spherical and is situated nearer the more rounded end. Towards the other end is a bluish stained body, the paranuclear body. The parasites multiply by longitudinal division; when multiplication occurs within a cell it becomes enlarged and packed with 'toxoplasms'[31]. These cells are referred to as pseudocysts; they have a distended cell membrane, the nucleus is pushed to the periphery and numerous parasites fill the cell. In chronic or inapparent infection 'pseudocysts' are invariably present.

Life cycle

The toxoplasm stage is an asexual stage in an intermediate host. This stage is probably transmitted to other animals also acting as intermediate hosts when infected muscle is ingested; transplacental infection of the foetus has also been recorded. However, when muscle containing toxoplasms is ingested by a cat, the parasite develops like a typical *Isospora* in the columnar cells of the intestine, and undergoes asexual and then sexual cycles. Oocysts are passed in the cat's faeces, and if the fully-developed oocysts are ingested by one of the many susceptible animals (including man) they develop as toxoplasms.

Mode of transmission

The mode of transmission of *T. gondii* from person to person is unknown except in congenital infections. Surveys of various populations have shown that a high incidence of asymptomatic infection occurs in the warm to hot humid areas, and a low incidence in the cold areas and hot dry areas. Serological tests in Singapore have shown that the Chinese—beef and pork eaters—have a lower frequency of antibodies to toxoplasmosis than Malays and Indians[32]. In general there does not appear to be any difference in infection rate between urban and rural populations, between sexes or between races in the same environment. *T. gondii* is widely distributed in the animal kingdom, being particularly common in cats, dogs and rabbits[33]. However, in spite of the circumstantial evidence indicating a possible transmission between animals and man, it is probable that both may become infected from a common source or sources. Ingestion of raw beef and pork meat is a recognized mode of infection and it has been demonstrated that infection was particularly high in a tuberculosis hospital in France, where the children were fed raw or underdone meat[34]. High infection ranges have also been found in sewage workers, rabbit trappers, laboratory workers, and nurses. The role of droplet infection, mechanical subcutaneous inoculation by biting, or bloodsucking arthropods in the transmission of toxoplasmosis has yet to be proved. Zigas and Benfante[35] have reviewed the whole subject and evaluated current progress in human toxoplasmosis. Roever-Bonnet[36] has reviewed the status of toxoplasmosis in seven African countries and it is clear that *T. gondii* is widely distributed in large parts of Africa, in man as well as animals.

Pathology

The infection may be congenital or acquired. The parasites proliferate in the cells of the reticuloendothelial system and parenchymal cells of practically every organ.

The most severe lesions are seen in striated muscle, the central nervous system, and heart. The lungs, liver, pancreas, spleen, testes, kidneys, hypophysis, and adrenal may also be affected and generalized lymphadenopathy is a feature of the more subacute form of the disease. The essential lesion in the acute form of the disease is a small area of focal necrosis surrounded by a variable cellular inflammatory reaction depending upon the tissue affected[37].

A focal embolic encephalomyelitis has been described in the brain but the usual changes are scattered small areas of focal necrosis surrounded by macrophages, lymphocytes and, occasionally, multinucleated giant cells. The Virchow-Robin space may be infiltrated with lymphocytes and plasma cells. Small pseudocysts may be seen in some foci and in other free toxoplasmas but usually there are no organisms. Pseudocysts may be present in the parenchymal cells with no surrounding reaction apparent.

In the myocardium pseudocysts are generally seen within the myofibrils and there are scattered foci of necrosis surrounded by monocytes and lymphocytes, with neutrophils and eosinophils present in variable numbers[38].

In the lungs non-specific bronchopneumonic changes may be found. An interstitial pneumonitis with proliferation of the alveolar lining cells, many containing parasites, and a gelatinous exudate in the alveoli are diagnostic if observed.

In striated muscle there is necrosis of individual fibres with sarcolemmal proliferation and infiltration around these necrotic areas by macrophages, lymphocytes and occasionally neutrophils. Once again pseudocysts may be seen in the muscle cells without a surrounding inflammatory reaction[39].

Lesions in the eye are usually unilateral but may be bilateral, and pathologically are most commonly diagnosed as tuberculosis or as a granulomatous lesion of unknown aetiology[40]. The retina, choroid, and frequently the sclera, are involved. There is necrosis of the retina and choroid with a surrounding zone of epitheloid cells and giant cells, some containing melanin pigment. Lymphocytes and plasma cells with varying numbers of eosinophils and neutrophils are also seen. Rounded structures containing amorphous eosinophilic material, possibly degenerate pseudocysts, may also be present in the necrotic material.

The glandular nodes show follicular hyperplasia with central chromatolysis. There is histiocytic proliferation in the sinusoids and islands of large eosinophilic histiocytic reticulum cells may be scattered throughout the gland. Foci of necrosis may be present. Parasites are rarely seen histologically although invariably isolated on animal inoculation[41].

Clinical features

Congenital toxoplasmosis is predominantly neurological, resulting from encephalomyelitis, the effects of which are evident at or soon after birth. Few infants survive the first few weeks of life, but some survive to adult life.

When the mother is infected early in pregnancy the usual effect on the foetus is hydrocephalus which commonly causes obstructed labour. Microcephalus may also occur. Infants who survive to childhood are mentally deficient and frequently suffer from epileptic convulsions. Ocular lesions, including vitreous opacities and choroidoretinitis, are common, and are associated with nystagmus. The characteristic retinal lesions are bilateral and lead to blindness; they are occasionally unilateral.

Micro-ophthalmia may be present in striking contrast to the enormous hydrocephalic head. Infection of the mother in the first trimester may also lead to abortion.

Acquired toxoplasmosis is usually divided into various clinical types, which are not separate entities but merely patterns determined by the site of the active infection.

Lymphatic toxoplasmosis is probably the commonest form of the infection. It is seen in patients of all ages, especially those concerned with domestic animals which may be reservoirs, such as pigs, cattle, dogs and rabbits. There is commonly generalized glandular enlargement, some groups of glands being more affected than others. The cervical, neck, axillary and inguinal glands are usually involved. The glands are discrete, moderately enlarged, firm but not tender, except during the febrile episodes which occur from time to time. The overlying skin is not involved. Mediastinal and pulmonary hilar glands are sometimes involved.

The glandular enlargement persists for months, sometimes for years. The spleen and liver are usually palpable.

Irregular moderate fever occurs in the early stages in many cases, usually starting before the appearance of the adenitis, and may persist for weeks, recurring at irregular intervals. Some cases are febrile throughout. The constitutional symptoms are commonly moderate, but may be severe.

The lymphatic syndrome is nearly always benign. The enlargement may last for years in children.

Cerebrospinal toxoplasmosis is commoner in children than in adults. The clinical picture is that of an acute or subacute meningoencephalitis. The onset is acute and in adults may be accompanied by a rash. There are fever, severe headache, cerebral vomiting, disorientation, delirium and sometimes maniacal attacks. Convulsions occur commonly in children. The patient often complains of rapidly advancing deafness and focal choroidoretinitis, which often involves the macula and eventually leads to scarring, visual disturbances and eventual blindness. Occasionally the attack is fulminating and death may occur in a few days from the onset. The course is usually a matter of months and in some cases, especially in adults, there are bouts of clinical signs of the meningoencephalitis with intervals of quiescence, sometimes extending over months or even years. Some patients recover without sequelae. Others have persistent headache and irregular explosions of maniacal or psychotic behaviour. In children the meningoencephalitis is usually fatal. In adults, recovery is common but there may be persistent neurological and psychotic sequelae. In some cases, the onset may take the form of suddenly developing abnormal behaviour and motor activity.

The cerebrospinal fluid is often xanthochromic, the protein content is considerably raised and leukocytes are present in large numbers.

Exanthematous toxoplasmosis occurs mainly in adults, usually individuals such as cattlemen closely concerned with reservoir animals. There is sudden onset with moderate to high fever, sometimes rigors. A generalized maculopapular erythematous rash develops after some days resembling the rash of tick typhus but absent from the palms and soles. Myalgia is present from the onset, with scattered areas of acutely painful localized tenderness, which persists after the acute phase has subsided, and may become palpable in the muscle substance.

There is commonly tachycardia and sometimes abnormal rhythms and cardiac dilatation. Pneumonitis develops in severe cases, with dyspnoea and sometimes respiratory failure. The syndrome may be complicated, especially in adults, with the signs of meningoencephalitis. Death may occur in the acute attack, or the disease may slowly devolve over some months.

Toxoplasmosis often exists without clinical expression and is discovered by laboratory tests.

Diagnosis

In the blood there may be a leukocytosis or leukopenia. An eosinophilia has been described[42]. There may be a mild degree of anaemia and a leukaemoid reaction and atypical lymphocytes may be seen.

Toxoplasma may be isolated from blood, cerebrospinal fluid, saliva, sputum, lymph nodes, skin, liver, and muscle by intraperitoneal injection of the biopsy or other material into mice, guinea-pigs, or hamsters. Mice are most suitable as they do not suffer from toxoplasmosis as a laboratory infection.

Histological examination of muscle (especially the gastrocnemius) or liver may reveal the presence of specific lesions, but the examination of lymph nodes usually fails to reveal the organisms although the pathology itself may point to a diagnosis. A portion of the biopsy should therefore not be put in fixative but should be refrigerated, and kept in a solution of penicillin and streptomycin, 100 units/ml of each in normal saline, prior to animal inoculation.

A number of serological tests have been described for the detection of antibodies to *T. gondii*; the cytoplasm-modifying test of Sabin-Feldman[43] (dye test) is the one most widely used. It is a sensitive test which shows the presence of antibody in many of the normal adult population; the most convincing method of diagnosing active toxoplasmosis is by the demonstration of at least a fourfold rise in titre, coupled with the isolation of toxoplasma in tissue or body fluids by inoculation of mice.

Other serological tests in common use are the complement fixation tests, direct agglutination test, haemagglutination test, and the fluorescent antibody test. Recently a toxoplasma neutralization test and a microagglutination test have been described. A review of the seroepidemiology of toxoplasma infection in man was given by Fleck[44].

Treatment

Pyrimethamine with or without sulphonamides is usually effective in acquired toxoplasmosis but the neurological sequelae resist treatment. Pyrimethamine is given in doses of 50 mg orally at once, followed in 6 hours by 25 mg. A dose of 25–50 mg is given daily for the next 13 days.

Sulphadiazine is given concurrently in doses of 1 g 6-hourly for 14 days. Sulphatriad 3 g immediately and 1 g 6-hourly may be used as an alternative.

Broad spectrum antibiotics including tetracycline and chlortetracycline have been used successfully, alone or with concurrent pyrimethamine, especially in heavy infections.

Folic acid and vitamin B are given concurrently. Thyroxin is sometimes given in addition. Corticosteroids have no effect on the acute stages of the disease, but may be given to relieve the neurological and psychotic effects; they have also been given for treatment for the choroidoretinitis, with equivocal results.

Some authors advise much longer treatment in severe intractable cases, continuing for several months on the same dose of pyrimethamine and 1–2 g sulphadiazine. This course puts a good deal of pressure on the bone marrow. Frequent white cell counts are necessary and the treatment should be interrupted for 2–3 weeks at intervals. The treatment is stopped if signs of bone marrow involvement appear.

Active infection in a woman in the first five months of pregnancy should be treated (short treatment). At this stage the infection may be stopped in the mother and congenital transmission may be prevented. If active disease is diagnosed later in pregnancy, the woman must again be treated, but the chances of congenital transmission may not be affected. A positive serum test before pregnancy without subsequent rise in titre indicates that treatment is unnecessary.

GIARDIA LAMBLIA

Giardia lamblia is a flagellate protozoa (Figure 7.3) belonging to the Superclass Mastigophora. The host–parasite relationship is very delicately balanced, often with host factors playing a dominant role in determining whether an infected person becomes ill or not.

Geographical distribution

Giardia lamblia, the cause of giardiasis, has a cosmopolitan distribution. In recent years several epidemics of symptomatic giardiasis have been noted: the

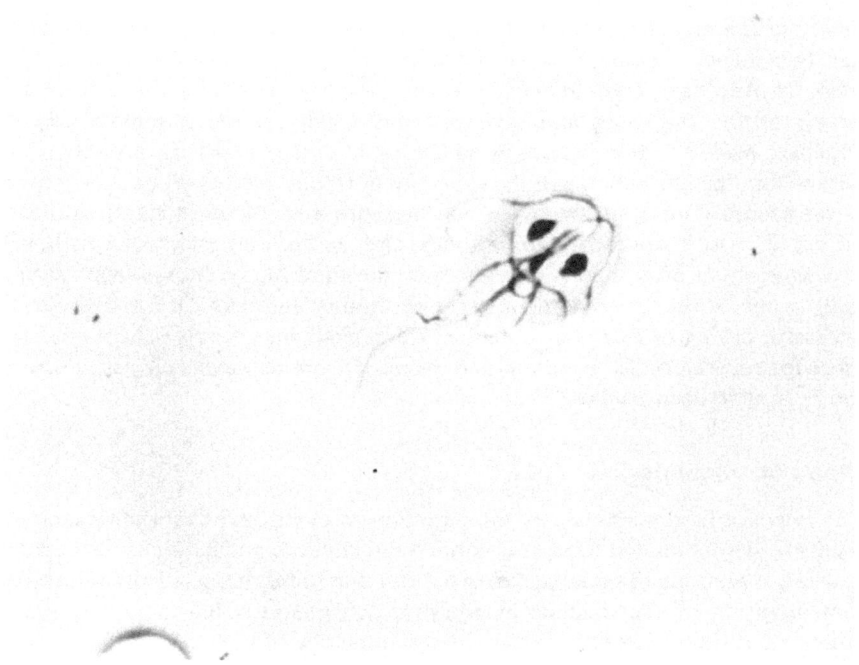

Figure 7.3 *Giardia lamblia*

first occurred in 1965–66 among skiers at Aspen, Colorado, and was traced to contamination of well water by sewage, whilst in 1972 a similar outbreak occurred in Boulder, Colorado, but the source was not discovered; in 1974 there were three recognized outbreaks in the USA that were traced in each case to contaminated drinking water. Visitors to endemic areas frequently become infected; many of the adults with symptomatic infections seen in Britain have recently returned from the tropics—persons travelling overland to India and Nepal are particularly affected. Similarly, American visitors to Russia, especially to Leningrad, have often become infected; a questionnaire survey of 1419 such persons showed that 23% had acquired giardiasis, and that attack rates were higher among those who had drunk tap water. In the United Kingdom in 1976 giardia was reported in 3051 cases[45–49].

Morphology and life cycle

The trophozoites of *Giardia lamblia* are pear-shaped discs that are pointed posteriorly; the mean dimensions are 15 μm in length, 9 μm in width and 3 μm in thickness. The dorsal surface is convex, while the ventral surface is flattened and bears a large sucking disc anteriorly, by which the organism attaches itself firmly to the mucosal surface of the jejunum and duodenum. The trophozoite has two nuclei, a centrally placed crescent-shaped parabasal body and four pairs of flagellae. Two axonemes (axostyles) run centrally throughout the length of the organism and give rise posteriorly to the hindmost pair of flagellae. Multiplication occurs by longitudinal binary fission. Encystation occurs within the gut lumen and the cysts are normally mature when they appear in the faeces. The cysts are ovoid and measure 8 to 14μm in length and 5 to 10 μm in width; there are four nuclei and up to four pairs of bristle-like axonemes may be visible. When there is intestinal hurry, motile trophozoites may occur in the stool, sometimes in enormous numbers. In the absence of excessive drying or extremes of temperature, cysts may survive in the environment for several weeks. Isolation and axenic culture as well as ultrastructure of the cyst have been studied[50,51].

Mode of transmission

The infection is transmitted by the ingestion of cysts, as a result of insanitary habits or contaminated food. It is common in children and in adults, sometimes causing symptoms of malabsorption in both due to mechanical irritation rather than invasion of the mucous membrane. *G. lamblia* is harboured by many animals but these play little part in the epidemiology of human infections. *Giardia* infections may persist for years and the parasite may invade the biliary tract. Symptomatic giardiasis is being increasingly recognized among travellers. During a 10-year study in India 23% of 300 patients with non-dysenteric diarrhoea were found to be infected with *Giardia*[52]. A 248-page monograph written in Rumanian has been devoted to giardiasis[53]. Of great interest is the relationship between *Giardia* infection and immunoglobulin deficiency syndromes[54]. A preponderance of blood group A has been found in Australian children with giardiasis.

Pathology

Histological studies of the jejunal and duodenal mucosa have been reported by many workers; frequently the findings have been correlated with absorption studies[55-59]. Symptomless subjects may show no mucosal abnormalities, but in patients with symptoms mild to severe partial villous atrophy may be seen, together with a quite extensive cellular infiltration of the lamina propria with lymphocytes, plasma cells and polymorphs. The crypts may be increased in length and show numerous mitoses. The villous epithelium is frequently cuboidal and may show extensive lymphocyte infiltration; Wright and Tomkins[60] have quantitated this infiltration and shown its correlation with clinical grading. Unlike coeliac patients, the epithelium in giardiasis often shows an increased number of goblet cells, together with well-preserved microvilli and basement membranes. When multiple biopsies are taken, a patchy distribution of mucosal abnormalities may be noted[61].

In sections parasites are normally seen adhering by their flattened ventral surfaces to the epithelium of the villi and crypts and this is likely to be their normal habitat. By the use of careful techniques mucosal invasion has been reported in several patients[62], and this has been confirmed in one subject by electron microscopy[63].

Most symptomatic patients show malabsorption of fat and D-xylose. Documentation of reduced folic acid and iron absorption is less clear; however, a reduced vitamin B_{12} absorption has been noted in some patients, as have low serum carotene levels[64]. Lactase deficiency is common in symptomatic subjects and may persist for considerable periods after treatment, especially in genetically predisposed individuals[65]. Barium studies normally reveal a non-specific malabsorption pattern.

Using *Giardia* cysts as antigen, Ridley and Ridley[66] have detected serum antibody by immunofluorescence in 32 of 36 cases of symptomatic giardiasis; there was some correlation between titre and the histological severity of jejunal lesions. Stools containing precystic or immature cyst forms provided the best antigen. Details of antigen preparation are given by Moody[67].

Several reports have shown an association between symptomatic giardiasis and immunodeficiency syndromes, in particular the relatively common non-selective variable hypogammaglobulinaemia.

The most common symptoms are poorly localized abdominal discomfort and distension, colic, borborygmi, flatulence and frequent loose, offensive and rather pale stools. Nausea, and sometimes heartburn or epigastric discomfort, is often noted after meals and may be followed by a diarrhoeal stool. The interval between infection and symptoms is commonly about 15 days; the illness may last for only a few days or may continue intermittently for two or three months. Symptoms are often worst at the beginning of the illness and may then subside spontaneously without treatment. The more severely affected can develop overt steatorrhoea and lose weight quickly, such patients show marked anorexia, malaise and lethargy.

Treatment

The most commonly used regimen in adults are mepacrine 100 mg t.d. for five to ten days, or metronidazole 250 or 400 mg t.d. for five to ten days[68]. Tinidazole (Fasigyn) at a dosage of 150 mg twice daily for seven days is also effective[69].

PLASMODIA

Of all the protozoan parasites that affect Western man, the plasmodia are by far the most important and of these *P. vivax* and *P. falciparum* are the ones most commonly encountered.

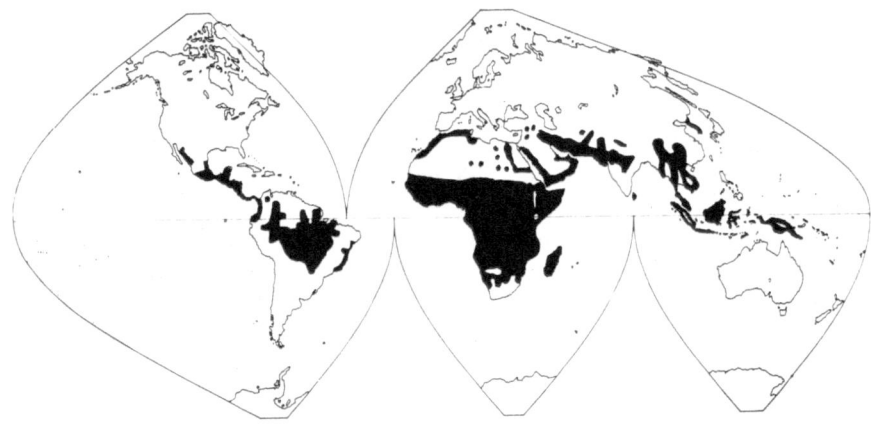

Figure 7.4   Map of malaria

Geographical distribution

The geographical distribution of the two parasites overlaps considerably and the malaria situation at the end of 1976 is given in Figure 7.4.

All the cases seen in Western Europe, America and Australasia are 'imported' and the figures available of the number of cases are shown in Tables 7.2 and 7.3.

Since 1967, a number of factors have adversely affected the progress of antimalaria activities in Asia, Central and South America and south-eastern Europe. Malaria epidemics have occurred in large areas previously freed from the disease. The main adverse factors are worldwide inflation, economic and energy crises, resistance of malaria vectors to current insecticides, high cost of alternative insecticides and chloroquine-resistant *P. falciparum* strains (Figure 7.5). In India 10 million cases of malaria have been reported in 1977 and in Pakistan 7 million cases.

Table 7.2   Cases of malaria imported into Europe (1976)

	P. vivax	*P. falciparum*
Bulgaria	40	16
Italy	34	67
Netherlands	36	30
Poland	12	5
Portugal	406	65
Spain	12	15
Yugoslavia	12	18

Table 7.3 Cases of malaria imported into England and Wales 1967–1977

	Notifications	Deaths
1967	111	4
1968	144	4
1969	124	8
1970	134	2
1971	240	9
1972	363	8
1973	447	3
1974	607	3
1975	601	5
1976	1162	3
1977	1477	9

Morphology and life cycle

The main morphological characters of the four human malaria species i.e. *P. vivax, P. falciparum, P. malariae* and *P. ovale* are given in standard textbooks of parasitology. The complete life cycle of the human malaria parasite embraces a period of development within the mosquito, and a period of infection in man.

After ingestion of human infected blood a period of development lasting 10–14 days occurs in the mosquito resulting in the production of sporozoites. A bite infects the human host with these forms, which remain in the circulating blood for 30 minutes or less then enter tissue cells notably in the liver, where the pre-erythrocytic cycle takes place.

During the succeeding 7–9 days the sporozoites develop in the parenchymal cells of the liver. This stage of development is known as the pre-erythrocytic

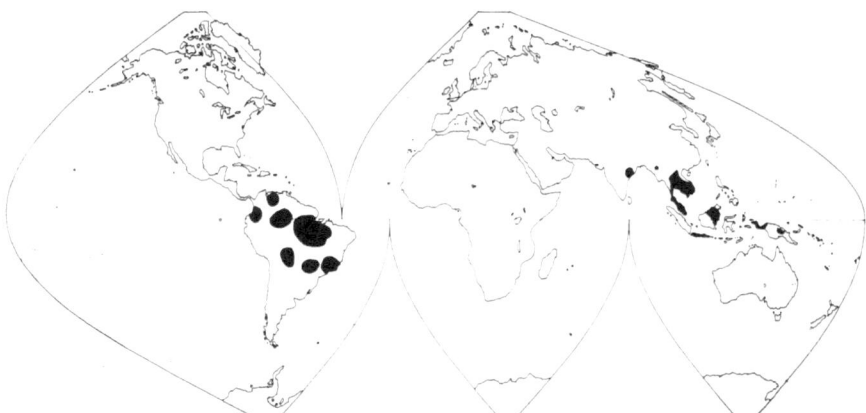

Figure 7.5 Map of chloroquine resistant malaria—here an extra blob should be added to New Guinea since chloroquine-resistant malaria now occurs both in West Irian as well as in Papua New Guinea proper

cycle. The cryptozoic schizonts thus formed rupture and release numerous merozoites, most of which enter the circulation to invade the erythrocytes, thus starting the erythrocytic cycle. Recent successful attempts at continuous culture[70] have led to the possibility of a malaria vaccine[71]. As in the short sporozoite phase no symptoms of malaria are experienced during the pre-erythrocytic cycle. Although Shortt and his colleagues[72] demonstrated pre-erythrocytic schizogony in human malaria in 1948, it is interesting to note that neither cryptozoic nor metazoic schizonts (exo-erythrocytic schizonts) have been reported in infections in man in areas of intense malaria transmission, despite search for these forms in liver biopsy and necropsy material. The liberation of the merozoites from the liver cells and their entry into the bloodstream initiates the erythrocytic cycle. The *Plasmodium* first appears in red cells as a small speck of chromatin surrounded by scanty cytoplasm, and soon becomes a ring-shaped trophozoite. As the parasite develops, pigment particles appear in the cytoplasm, and the chromatin is more prominent. Chromatin division then proceeds and when complete there is formed the mature schizont containing daughter merozoites. The parasitized red blood cell now ruptures, releasing merozoites, the majority of which re-enter erythrocytes to re-initiate erythrocytic schizogony. In *P. falciparum* infection the erythrocytic cycle takes 36–48 hours (subtertian); in *P. vivax* and *P. ovale* infection takes 48 hours (tertian) and in *P. malariae* 74 hours (quartan). The powers of invasion of the species of *Plasmodia* differ considerably. *P. vivax* develops most easily in the youngest erythrocytes, so that at any one time not more than 2% of red cells are invaded. *P. malariae* develops chiefly in the older red cells, the infection rate seldom exceeding 2%. In *P. falciparum* infection rates of up to 15%. or more of red cells have been noted, and preference for young cells has recently been demonstrated[73].

Much information is available regarding the metabolism of the malaria parasite from the moment it first invades the red blood cell to its subsequent development into a schizont. Both the metabolic pathways and nutritional requirement have been most extensively studied in avian malaria (*P. lophurae*). The malaria parasite appears to possess the same mechanism for the breakdown of glucose as its vertebrate host. The chief source of parasite protein is the haemoglobin of the erythrocyte. Electron microscopy studies have demonstrated that the parasites engulf portions of the red cell cytoplasm by invaginating their limiting membranes, a process known as 'phagotrophy'. The ultrastructure of red cells infected by *P. falciparum* in man was studied by Miller[74]. All available studies suggest that the nucleic acid metabolism of malaria parasites is similar to that of other organisms; moreover, it has been shown that malarial parasites have a very high lipid content. Several substances are needed for the extracellular survival of *P. lophurae*, e.g. pyruvate, diphosphopyridine nucleotide, adenosine triphosphate, malate, coenzyme A, leucovorin, red cell extract and gelatin[75]. These are probably also necessary for the development of malaria parasites of man. A detailed review of the metabolism of the malaria parasite and its host was carried out by Fletcher and Maegraith[76].

In response to some unknown stimulus a number of the merozoites released after erythrocytic schizogony develop into male and female forms known as gametocytes. Gametocytes are believed to be inert in man. They provide the reservoir of infection enabling mosquitoes to perpetuate the malaria cycle, and remain within the red cell for the duration of their survival, i.e. up to 120 days.

A certain proportion of the merozoites liberated from the cryptozoic schizonts of the pre-erythrocytic phase do not enter the bloodstream but re-enter the parenchymal cells of the liver to produce the secondary or metacryptozoic schizonts which are responsible for the persistence of the exo-erythrocytic (EE) cycle. The reappearance of malaria after clinical cure results from the parasite's ability to persist in the tissues in this EE form. The eventual discharge of merozoites from these EE forms into the bloodstream results in reinvasion of red blood cells, so producing a relapse. The exo-erythrocytic cycle occurs in *P. vivax, P. ovale* and *P. malariae* infections. *P. vivax* can usually produce relapses up to three years after infection; while *P. malariae* has occasionally relapsed 10, 20 or even 30 years after a primary infection. The existence of an exo-erythrocytic phase in *P. malariae* has recently been questioned (Garnham, personal communication). Patients suffering from *P. ovale* malaria have recently been seen in Europe and the United States of America. All the infections were contracted in West Africa and relatively long periods of latency were noticed. The infections were of considerable severity but spontaneous recovery was the rule. The mechanism of malaria relapse was studied by Contacos and Collins[77]. In *P. falciparum* malaria the liver phase is said not to persist; it follows therefore that when adequate treatment for the erythrocytic cycle is given relapses do not occur. It is therefore rare for *P. falciparum* infections to relapse after one year of freedom from exposure to infection, although a few authentic cases with long intervals prior to recrudescence have been described[78]. Enzyme typing of malaria parasites has demonstrated variations in *P. falciparum* in Gambia[79].

Mode of transmission

Malaria is transmitted by various species of *Anopheles* mosquitoes. Transmission, however, can also occur occasionally through blood transfusion—whole blood, plasma or platelets—and by syringe passage among drug addicts. In non-endemic areas 'air travel' is mostly responsible for the cases seen. Immunity to malaria has been reviewed by McGregor[80]. Miller[81] has shown that Duffy blood groups are involved in the racial immunity of negroes to *P. vivax* infection.

Pathology

Of the four malaria species, the only one which is directly fatal is *P. falciparum* and the pathology of malaria in the various organs refers mainly to the changes seen in *P. falciparum* infection[82].

The most severe lesions in the central nervous system occur in cerebral malaria. The meninges are grossly congested, the smaller vessels being packed with parasitized cells. The anaemia is often severe and haemolytic in origin. The bone marrow is greyish red, soft and hyperaemic and is increased in the long bones. In the acute stage its vessels are full of parasitized erythrocytes and haemozoin is present in the reticuloendothelial cells and monocytes. There is a marked normablastic hyperplasia even in the absence of a reticulocytosis in the peripheral blood and there is also myelocytic proliferation. In the acute attack the spleen is enlarged and tense, and the cut surface is slaty greyish red with the Malpighian corpuscles prominent. The consistency may be soft if a terminal bronchopneumonia is present. Histologically the blood vessels, Billroth cords and sinusoids are filled with parasitized red cells. Parasitized and unparasitized cells and haemozoin are seen in the pulp histiocytes and sinusoidal lining cells. Pigment may be found lying free in the pulp and sinusoids, and in our experience it is also found in the germinal follicles. A splenic smear reveals developing forms of parasites and haemozoin lying free and contained in monocytes. Degeneration of the endothelial cells of splenic vessels may occur causing thrombosis, haemorrhage and infarction.

With increasing immunity the spleen becomes at first jet black with much pigment in the cords, but gradually the congestion decreases and the pigment disappears first from the sinusoids and last from the cords with parasitized cells becoming scanty. The spleen diminishes in size, the capsule becomes greyish, fibrotic and wrinkled, perhaps with some evidence of long-standing perisplenitis, and some fibrosis is seen in the pulp.

The pathological changes in the liver vary according to the immunological status of the individual and the mode of death. In cerebral malaria the liver is enlarged and tense and its colour varies from dark red to slaty grey. If, however, anaemia has been gross the liver is enlarged and pale yellowish grey in colour.

Histologically the striking feature in the acute stage is the gross congestion of the sinusoids and centrilobular veins by parasitized erythrocytes. The Kupffer cells are hypertrophied and contain parasitized and unparasitized red blood cells, remnants of parasites and granules and masses of haemozoin, with haemosiderin inconstantly present. The parenchymal cells may contain haemosiderin but never haemozoin. One of the striking and constantly reported features has been degeneration and necrosis in the centrilobular regions in the absence of heart failure. The striking feature in the kidneys is gross congestion of the vessels with parasitized erythrocytes, especially in the capillaries of the glomerular tuft. Acute diffuse glomerulonephritis has been described in association with *P. falciparum* malaria. Tubular necrosis may occasionally occur. Changes in the adrenals are variable. Degenerative and necrotic changes in the inner zone of the cortex with loss of lipid have been described. The more usual finding, however, is gross congestion and haemorrhage.

Deaton[83] has described two patients dying of pulmonary oedema even though antimalarial therapy had cleared the parasitaemia and vigorous therapy was undertaken. The findings in the lung at autopsy in one case showed only pulmonary oedema with acute and subacute passive congestion. No parasitized erythrocytes were seen and no lesions were noticed in the heart or CNS to account for death. Overhydration did not appear to be a factor. Hyaline membrane formation, thickened alveolar septa and areas of alveolar haemorrhage have been noted in the lungs. The basic lesions appeared to be injury to the capillaries of the lung with congestion and leakage of oedema fluid.

Clinical features

The clinical pictures of P. vivax and P. falciparum are dealt with separately.

P. vivax

Fever is the most constant sign. After a brief period of remittent fever the pattern of intermittent regularly recurring fever every second day becomes established. The classical features of the attack—cold stage, hot stage, sweating stage—are unusual in infants and children. General symptoms similar to those described for P. falciparum infection may occur but are usually milder. The spleen enlarges early in the disease, some degree of anaemia may be present, and there is often mild leukopenia. Pernicious complications are rare, but if fever is high convulsions may occur in children. Vivax malaria per se is rarely lethal.

P. falciparum

There is little that is typical about falciparum malaria, and its many and various symptoms can be very misleading. A common misconception concerns the periodicity of the fever (Figure 7.6), which, especially in first attacks, is irregular and often of daily occurrence. Headache, malaise, nausea, vomiting and generalized joint pains may be the only additional presenting symptoms of an uncomplicated attack. On physical examination there may be hepatosplenomegaly, depending on how long the infection has been present, and a variable degree of anaemia. This rather undramatic clinical picture can deteriorate suddenly into one with severe manifestations where treatment may be hopeless.

Among these 'pernicious' manifestations the following are commonly recognized: cerebral malaria, renal insufficiency or failure, gastrointestinal malaria, algid malaria, malarial anaemia, hyperpyrexia, pulmonary oedema and malarial haemoglobinuria. Patients usually also have fever, show signs of dehydration, are moderately pale and may have Herpes labialis[84,85]. Jaundice with or without hepatic failure is a manifestation that is frequently misdiagnosed as infective hepatitis.

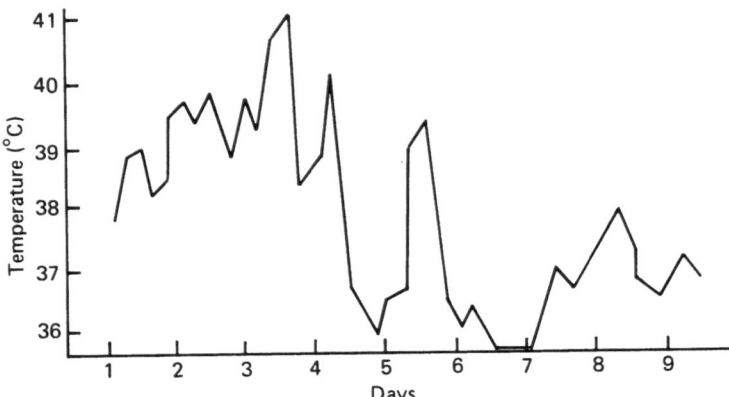

Figure 7.6   Temperature chart in *falciparum* malaria

Diagnosis

The only certain proof of the infection is the finding of malaria parasites in the peripheral blood and this examination should never be neglected. When malaria infection is causing severe clinical symptoms the diagnosis in most cases is clear after looking at only a few fields with an oil immersion lens. Usually the seriousness of the infection is proportional to the density of parasitaemia, but difficulty arises in the patient who has taken a small dose of an antimalarial drug, sufficient to clear most of the parasites from the peripheral blood but not to cure the infection.

The thick film gives better results in the hands of an experienced worker, but for the inexperienced the thin film is preferable. Some indication of density should be given since this is also useful as a measure of response to treatment. If rapid examination of blood films is not possible and the probability of malaria exists, adequate treatment must be instituted at once after taking the blood film, without waiting for its result.

Of the four parasite species, the invasive powers are greatest in *P. falciparum*, when 10% or more of the red cells may be parasitized. In *P. vivax* and *P. ovale* infection it is rare for more than 2% of erythrocytes to be invaded and in *P. malariae* 1% is exceptional. In blackwater fever malarial parasites are often scanty.

Treatment*

Irrespective of the species of *Plasmodium* the following oral regimen of chloroquine† will cure a clinical attack of malaria in chloroquine-sensitive areas:

---

* Children's dosages should be calculated according to the body surface area from existing tables
† There are several proprietary brands

Day 1. 600 mg (base) initially
       300 mg (base) 6 hours later
Day 2. 300 mg (base)
Day 3. 300 mg (base)

This regimen will produce a radical cure of *falciparum* malaria without relapses. On the other hand, for *P. vivax, P. malariae* and *P. ovale* this course of treatment must be combined with simultaneous administration of an 8-aminoquinoline (Primaquine or quinocide):

Chloroquine as above (3-day course) followed by
Primaquine 7.5 mg twice daily for 14 days

Certain strains of *P. vivax* (Chesson strain) from New Guinea require 21 days of Primaquine treatment instead of 14 days.

Severe and complicated attacks of *P. falciparum* require the use of parenteral antimalarials and equally important supportive medical treatment for the relevant complications.

The treatment of chloroquine-resistant *falciparum* malaria necessitates the use of quinine with sulfadoxine[86].

Although it is not absolutely necessary, individuals visiting or intending to reside in malarious areas should establish the prophylactic habit before they arrive. One of the following drugs should be taken *one week before arrival* and then *continuously throughout the period of exposure* and *for one month after leaving the endemic area*:

1. Proguanil hydrochloride (Paludrine) 100 mg (one 100 mg tablet) daily
2. Pyrimethamine (Daraprim) 25 mg (one 25 mg tablet) on the same day each week.
3. Chloroquine 300 mg (base) once a week.

Chemoprophylaxis in chloroquine-resistant areas is a difficult problem since in these areas *P. falciparum* is often also resistant to all other synthetic anti-malarial drugs. In the United Kingdom up-to-date advice should be sought from the specialized centres in Liverpool and London*.

PROTOZOA THAT ARE MAINLY CONFINED TO DEVELOPING COUNTRIES

The undermentioned protozoa only occasionally occur in the Western World and a very brief account of them will be given. For full details readers should consult other textbooks of human parasitology and tropical medicine (see 'Further Reading').

---

* At present 'Maloprim' (pyrimethamine and daprone), one tablet weekly is recommended

Trypanosoma

T. gambiense and *T. rhodesiense* are responsible for African sleeping sickness. They occur within a wide belt of territory in Africa stretching from Senegal and southern Sudan in the north to Angola and Portuguese East Africa in the south. Regions of very high endemicity occur in Guinea, Ghana, Nigeria, Gambia, Sierra Leone and Zaire. It is estimated that in Africa there are about 35 million people at risk[87]. In the Western world infection is occasionally seen in travellers and tourists to safari parks (Figure 7.7).

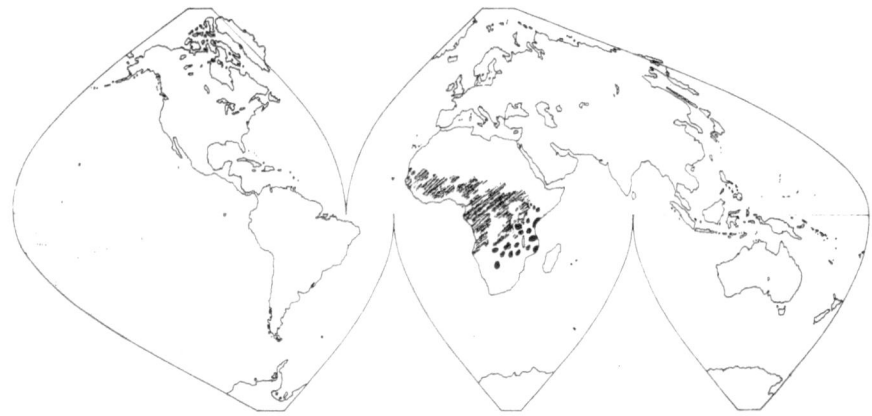

Figure 7.7   Map of African trypanosomiasis

In man *T. gambiense* and *T. rhodesiense* are morphologically identical. They appear in the blood tissue fluids as thin slender flagellates (trypomastigotes) (Figure 7.8) 10–30 μm in length; when various species of *Glossina* (tsetse fly) bite, the trypomastigotes are taken with the blood into the mid-gut and multiply. The most important species of *Glossina* are *G. palpalis*, *G. pallipides*, *G. tachinoides* and *G. morsitans*. The fly becomes infective 18–34 days after feeding on blood containing trypanosomes.

In *gambiense* trypanosomiasis pathological changes develop at the site of the injection of the parasite, in the bloodstream, in the lymphatic and connective tissues, in certain visceral organs including the heart, and at a later stage, in the central nervous system especially the brain and to some extent the cord with accompanying changes in the cerebrospinal fluid.

In *rhodesiense* trypanosomiasis the pathology is essentially the same but involvement of lymphatic glands is less common and by the time of death the involvement of the central nervous system is frequently not as fully advanced as in *gambiense* infection. In *rhodesiense* infections, serous effusions are more common and lesions in the heart more frequent and severe.

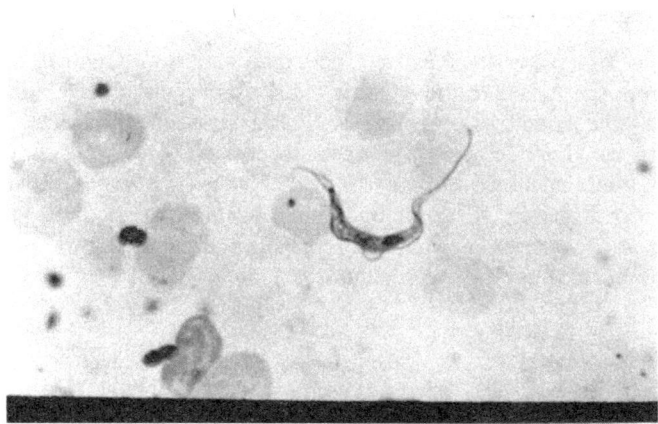

Figure 7.8 Trypanosome in blood

The classical clinical picture of *gambiense* trypanosomiasis can be divided into several stages. First, there is the tumour at the site of the bite. Then follows the stage of invasion, starting as a septicaemia succeeded after a variable interval by invasion of the lymph glands. This in turn is followed by nervous system involvement. The progress of the disease occupies anything from nine months to three years or more from the first appearance of symptoms.

In *rhodesiense* infection the local reaction at the bite is often severe. The incubation period may be shorter than in *gambiense* infections. The disease may start with rigor and severe fever. The lymph glands are commonly little involved although there may be some enlargement in the glands of the posterior triangle of the neck. Trypanosomes appear earlier in the blood and in larger numbers than in corresponding *gambiense* infections. Scattered fleeting firm oedematous subcutaneous swellings may occur. There is acute loss of weight and emaciation. The clinical signs of cardiac involvement appear early. The pulse is fast from the onset and remains so even in remissions; cardiac dilatation and incompetence are common. The central nervous system is involved early, sometimes within 4–5 weeks of the onset, but the meningoencephalitic processes are seldom as advanced at death as those of *gambiense* trypanosomiasis, possibly because of the shorter duration of the disease. Mental symptoms, especially progressive delusional states, are usual.

Diagnosis of trypanosomiasis depends on the discovery of the parasite. Search for the organism may be made in the blood, glandular juice and cerebrospinal fluid. Fluid from the bite tumour taken within two days of infection usually contains parasites. The ELISA technique has also been used in the diagnosis of trypanosomiasis[88].

Drugs commonly used for the treatment of trypanosomiasis are suramin, pentamidine, melarsoprol and nitrofurazone. Prophylaxis against *T. gambiense* is feasible using pentamidine or suramin.

Chagas' disease

Chagas' disease exists in localized endemic zones in Central and South America from the Andes to the Atlantic coast as far south as the latitude of the River Plate. The causative organism is *T. cruzi*. It occurs characteristically in blood films as short 'c'- or 's'-shaped trypomastigotes with a prominent kinetoplast. Reduvid bugs particularly in the genera *Triatoma, Rhodnius* and *Panstrongylus* transmit *T. cruzi* by faecal contamination. The infection is characterized by local oedema, myocardial changes, cardiomegaly and enteromegaly. Treatment is unsatisfactory[89].

Leishmania

A number of species belonging to the genus *Leishmania* are responsible for the various manifestations of leishmaniasis. A recent classification is given in Table 7.1.

As an unfortunate sequel to the breakdown of malaria control in India, there has developed an epidemic of visceral leishmaniasis in the State of Bihar affecting over 100 000 people. In the Western world most cases of visceral leishmaniasis are acquired by people enjoying a holiday in the countries bordering the Mediterranean or in immigrants from endemic areas. There were three infections with *Leishmania* species in the United Kingdom in 1976.

This genus occurs in man in the amastigote form only. The parasite has a body of round or oval shape which measures about 2 to 5 μm in size and it contains two structures easily visible in stained preparations. The first is the nucleus, which is a large, round or oval, solid-looking structure; the second is the kinetoplast, which is usually rod-shaped and which, though considerably smaller than the nucleus, is more deeply stained.

Visceral leishmaniasis (Kala-azar)

This condition is very widespread (Figure 7.9) and occurs in four main epidemiological forms depending on the geographical area concerned, i.e. Indian Kala-azar, Mediterranean Kala-azar, African Kala-azar and South and Central American Kala-azar. Thus, it is found in India, central Asia, China, Sudan, tropical Africa and South America. A large epidemic occurred in 1974–77 in Bihar State, India, involving around 100 000 cases and about 4000 deaths.

Leishmania donovani parasitizes reticuloendothelial cells and is found in greatest numbers in those organs which are particularly rich in this tissue. Its presence leads to great proliferation of macrophage-type cells. Histologically the outstanding feature of parasitized tissue is the enormous proliferation of cells of the macrophage type; their presence overshadows the normal structure of the organ, and many of the macrophages in the tissue will be seen to contain *Leishmania*.

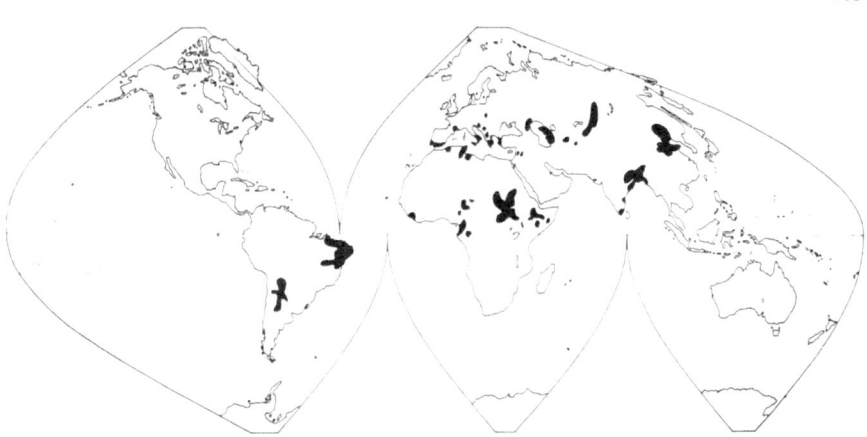

Figure 7.9   Map of visceral leishmaniasis

The outstanding physical signs are progressive enlargement of the spleen and, to a lesser extent, of the liver. The fever, which is intermittent, remittent, or continuous, recurs irregularly. The patient is rarely prostrated, and does not usually suffer from the subjective symptoms of fever. Delirium, even in the last stages of the disease, is unusual. The temperature at some time during the course of a febrile attack may show a double, or a treble, diurnal rise to high peaks (Figure 7.10). There is often a leukopenia.

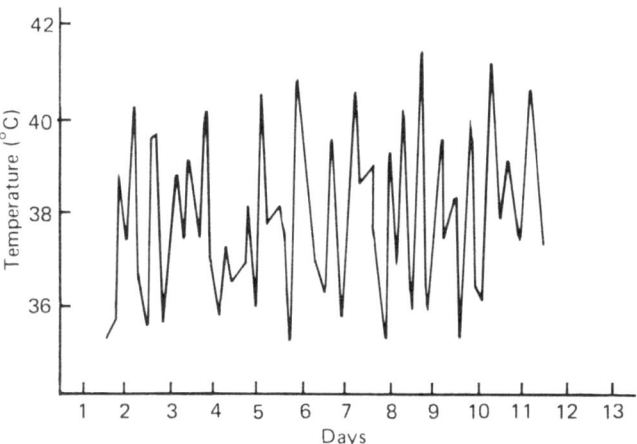

Figure 7.10   Temperature chart in visceral leishmaniasis

Diagnosis is established as follows:

(i) By examination of stained films of peripheral blood.

(ii) Culture of the peripheral blood, or of blood from a vein, is frequently successful when microscopic examination fails to reveal parasites.

(iii) Examination of juice obtained from gland puncture is sometimes successful in Indian infections.

(iv) Puncture of the sternum for marrow smears is considered good and safer than spleen puncture. Puncture of the tibia in children is also recommended. If hamsters are available they should be inoculated with 1 to 5 ml quantities of blood, or bone marrow.

(v) Examination of scrapings of sections of the skin lesions in dermal leishmanoids may reveal free and intracellular parasites.

Pentavalent antimonials, e.g. urea stibamine and sodium stibogluconate (Pentostam) are the drugs of choice. The diamidines are also effective.

Naegleria

Since 1958 there have been about 40 recorded cases of human infection with amoebae which are normally free-living. At first these amoebae were thought to be *Acanthamoeba*, but recent work suggests that only a single species of *Naegleria*, *N. aerobia*, is involved. When in man, these amoebae produce an infection resembling a fulminating bacterial meningitis, which has been given the name of 'primary amoebic meningoencephalitis', with a sudden onset of symptoms usually causing death within one week. Infections are frequently associated with swimming in small bodies of fresh water, especially those polluted with sewage. Infection of man seems to occur following contamination of the nasal mucosa with amoebic trophozoites, which penetrate through the mucous membrane and invade the brain via the olfactory bulbs. No satisfactory treatment for this infection has been found.

Isospora belli

The oocyst is ovoid in shape, 23 to 33 μm long and 12 to 14 μm wide, with a moderate neck-like narrowing at one end; the cyst wall is thin and translucent. Fresh cysts contain a large central spherical granular mass containing the nucleus; on further development the central mass divides into two daughter cells or sporoblasts that secrete cell walls to become spherical sporocysts within the oocyst wall. Each sporoblast then undergoes two nuclear divisions to form four crescent-shaped, uninucleate sporozoites within each spherical sporocyst.

I. belli is usually reported from the tropics, but may also be common in mental institutions[90] and other situations that favour faeco-oral transmission[91]. While some *I. belli* infections are symptomless, it is clear from reports of accidental infections, experimental infections and detailed case reports that this organism can cause significant disease[92].

The most frequent symptoms are colicky abdominal pain, flatulence and diarrhoea; the stools are often pale and may contain mucus and undigested food; malaise and anorexia are common and there may be low fever. Symptoms rarely last more than two or three weeks, but in the most severe cases a prolonged syndrome resembling sprue or coeliac disease may be produced with considerable weight loss. Jarpa Gana[93] has described a personal series of 57 patients from Chile, most of whom had symptoms including diarrhoea, weight loss and fever; illnesses lasted for six weeks to six months. Treatment is unsatisfactory.

Isospora hominis

The faecal forms of this parasite are more mature than those of *I. belli* and have normally lost their oocyst wall. Typically they appear as single or paired sporocysts that are ovoid in shape (mean length $14 \mu m$) and contain four sporozoites. It is now believed that the sporocysts are not infective for man but must be ingested by cattle or pigs for the cycle to continue. It has been shown experimentally[94] that man becomes infected by eating uncooked beef or pork containing sarcocysts that are visible macroscopically as minute greyish-white streaks.

The distribution of *I. hominis* is more localized and it is not normally found in mental hospitals or military barracks. Careful searches may reveal high rates of infection, for example 7% or more in Holland, and 10–60% in Kenya. Infection rates are related to the local dietary custom of eating improperly cooked meat.

Most reports of *I. hominis* infections describe either mild self-limiting gastrointestinal symptoms or none at all.

Balantidium coli

The trophozoite of *Balantidium coli* is an oval and flattened ciliate protozoon measuring from 50 to 100 μm in length by 50 to 70 μm in breadth. It produces rounded cysts, measuring about 50 μm in diameter, which are passed in the stools. The parasite is a common one of pigs, and occurs also in guinea pigs, monkeys and in man.

Many mammals are naturally infected but it is believed that the pig and, less commonly, the rat are the common sources of infection in man. Pigs all over the world are infected, including about 80% of those in the United Kingdom. Human infection is often common where human contact with pigs is particularly close, as in New Guinea, Micronesia, southern Russia and parts of south and central America. However, human infections also occur in Moslem countries and in mental institutions, and in such circumstances person to person transmission is probably important. In temperate countries the infection is exceedingly rare in man.

Most infections in man are asymptomatic and it has been suggested that debility, intercurrent disease or malnutrition is necessary for tissue invasion to occur[95]. Children appear to be more susceptible than adults. In pigs, *Salmonella* infection and whipworm (*Trichuris*) encourage tissue invasion; similar factors may operate in man, in particular *Trichuris* infection[96].

Symptomatology is very similar to that of invasive amoebiasis but with a greater tendency in severe cases to bowel perforation. Mild cases may present themselves as intermittent diarrhoea; in such patients at least some of the stools passed will normally be blood-stained.

Unformed or dysenteric stools contain only trophozoites; in formed stools there may be both cysts and trophozoites. Under suitable conditions trophozoites can persist in the environment for 24 hours or more. In fresh wet preparations recognition of motile trophozoites is easy, but in preserved specimens they may be overlooked. Cysts are usually rather scanty in human stools and their presence may be intermittent; unless concentration techniques are used for the detection of carriers, many will be missed. Trophozoites may also be found in scrapings from ulcers seen at endoscopy.

Tetracycline is the treatment of choice while metronidazole has been reported effective in a small series of patients from Venezuela.

Trichomonas

T. hominis inhabits the caecum and large intestine. The body is pear-shaped, 8–15 μm in length. The single ovoid nucleus is situated in the rounded anterior end and there are three flagella. There is no cystic phase. The presence of these flagellates in diarrhoeic stools has no pathogenic significance. *T. vaginalis* is found in the vagina and male urethra. It is larger than *T. hominis*, reaching 27 μm in length, and usually has five anterior flagella. No cysts are known. The flagellate is commonly found during the reproductive period in women, and men play an important part in the transmission of the infection. The incidence of infection in the vagina may be high and the presence of the parasite is associated with lowered vaginal acidity.

In the female vaginitis is usual and an anterior urethritis may occur. Posterior urethritis is rare and the bladder is never affected.

The vagina is inflamed and tender. Erosions may be present which histologically show a superficial coagulum containing trichomonads and cellular elements of the blood. In the submucosa there is a non-specific chronic inflammatory reaction with a variable number of neutrophil polymorphonuclears present. Trichomonads may or may not be seen. Secondary infection is usual in these cases.

In the male urethritis is not uncommon and the infection may spread to the bladder and prostate gland. The condition is usually mild unless secondary infection occurs.

Diagnosis is made by finding the flagellate in vaginal and prostatic secretions or in the urine. *T. vaginalis* may be identified in the moist slide by dark ground or phase contrast microscopic examination. Inoculation of a vaginal swab into culture medium incubated at 37 °C for 24–48 hours will give better results. The organism may also be identified in cervical smears stained by the Papanicolaou method.

Babesia

Piroplasms are widely distributed in cattle and dogs, their presence may present a hazard to splenectomized persons or to those whose splenic or immunological function is deficient[97] (see Chapter 9).

References

1. Poltera, A. A. (1973). Pseudomalignant cutaneous amoebiasis in Uganda. *Trop. Geogr. Med.*, **25**, 139
2. Cooke, R. A (1973). Cutaneous amoebiasis involving the anogenital region. *J. Med. Ass. Thailand*, **56**, 354
3. Sepulveda, B. and Diamond, L. S. (1976). Proceedings of the International Conference on Amoebiasis, Mexico City. October 27–29, 1975. Instituto Mexicano del Seguro Social, Mexico
4. Neal, R. A. and Harris, W. G. (1975). Attempts to infect inbred strains of rats and mice with *Entamoeba histolytica*. *Trans. R. Soc. Trop. Med. Hyg.*, **69**, 429
5. Griffin, J. L. (1972). Human amoebic dysentery. Electron microscopy of *Entamoeba histolytica* contacting, ingesting and digesting inflammatory cells. *Am. J. Trop. Med. Hyg.*, **21**, 895
6. Takeuchi, A. and Phillips, B. P. (1975). Electron microscope studies of experimental *Entamoeba histolytica* infection in the guinea pig. I. Penetration of the intestinal epithelium by trophozoites. *Am. J. Trop. Med. Hyg.*, **24**, 34
7. Takeuchi, A. and Phillips, B. P. (1976). Electron miscroscope studies of experimental *Entamoeba histolytica* infection in the guinea pig. II. Early cellular and vascular changes accompanying invasion in the lamina propria. *Virchows Archiv. B. Zell. Pathologie*, **20**, 87
8. Diamond, L. S. and Mattern, C. F. T. (1976). Protozoal viruses. *Adv. Virus Res.*, **20**, 87
9. Henley, G. L., Lee, C. M. and Takeuchi, A. (1976). Freeze-etching observations of trophozoites of pathogenic *Entamoeba histolytica*. *Z. Parasit.*, **48**, 181
10. Knight, R. (1975). Surveys for amoebiasis. Interpretation of data and their implications. *Ann. Trop. Med. Parasite.*, **69**, 35
11. Ross, G. W. and Knight, R. (1973). Dietary factors affecting the pathogencity of *Entamoeba histolytica* in rats. *Trans. R. Soc. Trop. Med. Hyg.*, **67**, 560
12. Knight, R. and Warren, K. S. (1973). The interaction between *Entamoeba histolytica* and *Schistosoma mansoni* infections in mice. *Trans. R. Soc. Trop. Med. Hyg.*, **67**, 644
13. Knight, R. and Chew, L. H. (1974). The interaction between *Entamoeba histolytica* and *Trichuris muris* infections in mice. *Am. J. Trop. Med. Hyg.*, **23**, 590
14. Edington, G. M. and Gilles, H. M. (1976). *Pathology in the Tropics.* 2nd Ed. 951 p. (London: Edward Arnold)
15. Quenum, C., Ndiaye, P. D. and Bayo, S. (1975). A study of 92 cases of malignant amoebic colitis. *Bull. Soc. Med. Afr. Noire Lang. Fr.*, **20**, 367 (in French)
16. Ramachandran, S., De Saram, R., Rajapakse, C. N. A. and Siralingham, S. (1973). Hepatic manifestations during amoebic dysentery. *Postgrad. Med. J.*, **49**, 261
17. Anh, D. H. (1971). Amoebic granuloma of the colon; a histopathological study of four cases. *S. E. Asian J. Trop. Med. Publ. Hlth.*, **2**, 34

18. Adams and Maegraith (1976). *Clinical Tropical Diseases.* 6th Ed. 592 p. (Blackwell Scientific Publications)
19. Rasaretnam, R. and Wijetilake, S. E. (1976). Left lobe amoebic liver abscess. *Postgrad. Med. J.,* **52,** 269
20. Ramachandran, S. (1974). Radiological changes in left lobe amoebic liver abscesses. *Postgrad. Med. J.,* **50,** 689
21. Stamm, W. P., Ashley, M. J. and Bell, K. (1976). The value of amoebic serology in an area of low endemicity. *Trans. R. Soc. Trop. Med. Hyg.,* **70,** 49
22. Stamm, W. P. and Phillips, E. A. (1977). A cellulose acetate membrane precipitin (CAP) test for amoebiasis. *Trans R. Soc. Trop. Med. Hyg.,* **71,** 490
23. Krupp, I. M. (1974). Comparison of counter-immunoelectrophoresis with other serologic tests in the diagnosis of amebiasis. *Am. J. Trop. Med. Hyg.,* **23,** 27
24. Alper, E. I., Littler, C. and Monroe, L. S. (1976). Counter-electrophoresis in the diagnosis of amebiasis. *Am. J. Gastroenterol.,* **65,** 63
25. Bos, H. J., Van der Eijk, A. A. and Steerenberg. P. A. (1976). Application of ELISA—enzyme-linked immunosorbent assay in the diagnosis of amoebiasis. *Trans. R. Soc. Trop. Med. Hyg.,* **69,** 440
26. Viana, R. L., Rego, A. and Antunes Dias, F. A. (1974). Amoebic abscess of the liver: scanning and selective hepatic arteriography. *S. Afr. Med. J.,* **48,** 96
27. Bieler, E. U., Meyer, B. J., Jensen, C. R. and Du Toit, D. (1974). The liver in amoebic disease. A report on clinical and scintiographic observations in 247 patients. *S. Afr. Med. J.,* **48,** 308
28. Matthews, A. E., Gough, K. R., Davies, E. R., Ross, F. G. M. and Hinchliffe, A. (1973). The use of combined ultrasonic and isotope scanning in the diagnosis of amoebic liver disease. *Gut,* **14,** 50
29. Chowcat, N. L. and Wyllie, J. H. (1976). Intravenous metronidazole in amoebic enterocolitis. *Lancet,* **ii,** 1143
30. Scragg, J. N., Rubidge, C. J. and Proctor, E. M. (1976). Tinidazole in treatment of acute amoebic dysentery in children. *Arch. Dis. Childh.,* **51,** 385
31. Zaman, V. and Colley, F. C. (1972). Ultrastructural study of penetration of macrophages by *Toxoplasma gondii. Trans. Roy. Soc. Trop. Med. Hyg.,* **66,** 781
32. Zaman, V. and Goh, T. K. (1969). Toxoplasmic antibodies in various ethnic groups in Singapore. *Trans. Roy. Soc. Trop. Med. Hyg.,* **63,** 884
33. Hutchison, W. M. (1972). Cats as a source of toxoplasmosis. *Proc. Roy. Soc. Med.,* **65,** 1001
34. Desmonts, G., Couvreur, J., Aliston, F., Baudelot, J., Gerbeaux, J. and Lelong, M. (1965). Étude épidémiologique sur la toxoplasmose: de l'influence de la cuisson des viandes de boucherie sur la fréquence de l'infection humaine. *Rev. Franç. Etude Clin. Biol.,* **10,** 952
35. Zigas, V. and Benfante, R. J. (1972). Human toxoplasmosis: an evaluation of current progress. *Trop. Geogr. Med.,* **24,** 1
36. Roever-Bonnet, H. de. (1972). Toxoplasmosis in tropical Africa. *Trop. Geogr. Med.,* **24,** 7
37. Remington, J. S., Jacobs, L. and Kaufman, H. E. (1960). Toxoplasmosis in the adult. *N. Engl. J. Med.,* **262,** 180
38. Sexton, R. C., Eyles, D. E. and Dillman, R. E. (1953). Adult toxoplasmosis. *Am. J. Med.,* **14,** 366
39. Chander, K., Mair, H. J. and Mair, N. S. (1968). Case of *Toxoplasma polymyositis. Br. Med. J.,* **1,** 158
40. Wilder, H. C. (1952). *Toxoplasma* chorioretinitis in adults. *A.M.A. Arch. Ophthalmol.,* **48,** 127
41. Saunders, S. J. and Thatcher, G. N. (1963). Toxoplasmosis in the adult. *S. Afr. Med. J.,* **37,** 1026
42. Cathie, I. A. B. (1954). *Toxoplasma* adenopathy in a child with isolation of the parasite. *Lancet,* **ii,** 115
43. Sabin, A. B. and Feldman, H. A. (1948). Dyes as microchemical indicators of a new immunity phenomenon affecting a protozoon parasite (*Toxoplasma*). *Science, N.Y.* **108,** 660
44. Fleck, D. (1972). The seroepidemiology of toxoplasma infection in man. *Proc. Roy. Soc. Med.,* **65,** 1002
45. Leading Article. (1974). Epidemic giardiasis. *Lancet,* **ii,** 1493

46. Thompson, R. G., Karandikan, D. S. and Leak, J. (1974). Giardiasis: an unusual cause of epidemic diarrhoea. *Lancet,* i, 615
47. Barbour, A. G., Nichols, C. R. and Kukushima, T. (1976). An outbreak of giardiasis in a group of campers. *Am. J. Trop. Med. Hyg.,* 25, 384
48. Brady, P. G. and Wolfe, J. C. (1974). Waterborne giardiasis. *Ann. Int. Med.,* 81, 498
49. Brodsky, R. E., Spencer, H. C. Jr. and Schultz, M. G. (1974). Giardiasis in American travellers to the Soviet Union. *J. Infect. Dis.,* 130, 319
50. Meyer, E. A. (1976). *Giardia lamblia:* Isolation and axenic culture. *Exp. Parasitol.,* 39, 101
51. Sheffield, H. G. and Bjorvatn, B. (1977). Ultrastructure of the cyst of *Giardia lamblia. Am. J. Trop. Med. Hyg.,* 26, 23
52. Antia, F. P., Desai, H. G., Jeejeebhoy, K. N., Kane, M. P. and Borkar, V. V. (1966). Giardiasis in adults: incidence, symptomatology and absorption studies. *Ind. J. Med. Sci.,* 20, 471
53. Lucian, O. (1971). *Lambliaza.* Editura Academiei Republicii Socialiste, Romania, Bucharest.
54. Brown, W. R. *et al.* (1972). Clinical, microbiological and immunnological studies in patients with immunoglobulin deficiences and gastrointestinal disorders. *Gut,* 13, 441
55. Yardley, J. H., Takano, J. and Hendrix, T. P. (1964). Epithelial and other mucosal lesions of jejunum in giardiasis. Jejunal biopsy studies. *Bull. Johns Hopkins Hosp.,* 115, 389
56. Hoskins, L. C., Winawer, S. J., Broitman, S. A., Gothlieb, L. S. and Zamcheck, N. (1967). Clinical giardiasis and intestinal malabsorption. *Gastroenterol.,* 53, 265
57. Tewan, S. G. and Tandon, B. N. (1974). Functional and histological changes of small bowel in patients with *Giardia lamblia* infestation. *Ind. J. Med. Res.,* 62, 689
58. Ridley, M. J. and Ridley, D. S. (1976). Serum antibodies and jejunal histology in giardiasis associated with malabsorption. *J. Clin. Pathol.,* 29, 30
59. Wright, S. G., Tomkins, A. M. and Ridley, D. S. (1977). Giardiasis. Clinical and therapeutic aspects. *Gut,* 18, 343
60. Wright, S. G. and Tomkins, A. M. (1977a). Quantitation of the lymphocyte infiltrate in jejunal epithelium in giardiasis. *Clin. Exp. Immunol.* (In press)
61. Ament, M. E. and Rubin, C. E. (1972). Relation of giardiasis to abnormal intestinal structure and function in gastrointestinal immunodeficiency syndromes. *Gastroenterol.,* 62, 216
62. Brandborg, L. L., Tankersley, C. B., Gottlieb, S., Barancik, M. and Santor, V. E. (1967). Histological demonstration of mucosal invasion by *Giardia lamblia* in man. *Gastroenterol.,* 52, 143
63. Morechi, R. and Parker, J. G. (1967). Ultrastructural studies of the human *Giardia lamblia* and subjacent jejunal mucosa in a subject with steatorrhoea. *Gastroenterol.,* 52, 151
64. Ember, M. and Mindszenty, L. (1969). Effect of giardiasis upon vitamin A metabolism. *Parasitologia,* 2, 55
65. Wolfe, M. S. (1975). Giardiasis. *J. Am. Med. Assoc.,* 233, 1362
66. Ridley, M. J. and Ridley, D. S. (1976). Serum antibodies and jejunal histology in giardiasis associated with malabsorption. *J. Clin. Pathol.,* 29, 30
67. Moody, A. H. (1976). Improved method for the pure preparation of faecal cysts for use as antigen. *Trans. R. Soc. Trop. Med. Hyg.,* 70, 338
68. Knight, R. (1978). Giardiasis, Isosporiasis and Balantidiasis. *Clin. Gastroenterol.,* 7, 31
69. Green, E., Lynch, D. M., McFadzean, J. A. and Pugh, I. M. (1976). Treatment of giardiasis. *Br. Med. J.,* 3, 411
70. Trager, W. and Jensen, J. B. (1976). Human malaria parasites in continuous culture. *Science (Washington),* 193, 673
71. Symposium on prospects for malaria vaccines. (1977). *Trans. R. Soc. Trop. Med. Hyg.,* 71, 4.
72. Shortt, H. E. and Garnham, P. C. C. (1948). The pre-erythrocytic development of *Plasmodium cynomolgi* and *Plasmodium vivax. Trans. R. Soc. Trop. Med. Hyg.,* 41, 785
73. Pasvol, G., Weatherall, D. J., Wilson, R. J. M., Smith, D. H. and Gilles, H. M. (1976). *Lancet,* i, 1269
74. Miller, L. H. (1972). The ultrastructure of red cells infected by *Plasmodium falciparum* in man. *Trans. R. Soc. Trop. Med. Hyg.,* 66, 3
75. Trager, W. (1958). Folinic acid and non-dialysable materials in the nutrition of malaria parasites. *J. Exp. Med.,* 108, 753

76. Fletcher, K. A. and Maegraith, B. G. (1972). The metabolism of the malaria parasite and its host. *Adv. Parasitol.*, **10**, 31
77. Contacos, P. G. and Collins, W. E. (1973). Malaria relapse mechanism. *Trans. R. Soc. Trop. Med. Hyg.*, **4**, 617
78. Verdrager, J. (1964). Observations on the longevity of *Plasmodium falciparum*: with special reference to findings in Mauritius. *Bull. Wld. Hlth. Org.*, **31**, 747
79. Carter, R. and McGregor, I. A. (1973). A. Enzyme variation in *Plasmodium falciparum* in the Gambia. *Trans. R. Soc. Trop. Med. Hyg.*, **67**, 830
80. McGregor, I. A. (1974). Immunity and malaria in man. *Tropical Doctor*, **4**, 104
81. Miller, L. H., Mason, S. J., Clyde, D. F. and McGinniss, M. H. (1976). The resistance factor to *Plasmodium vivax* in blacks. The Duffy-blood-group genotype, *Fyfy*. *N. Engl. J. Med.*, **295**, 302
82. Edington, G. M. and Gilles, H. M. (1976). *Pathology in the Tropics*. 2nd Edition. 951 pp. (London: Edward Arnold)
83. Denton, J. G. (1970). Fatal pulmonary oedema as a complication of acute falciparum malaria. *Am. J. Trop. Med. Hyg.*, **19**, 196
84. Gilles, H. M. (1976). Malaria. (Symposium Royal College of Physicians, Edinburgh)
85. Harinasuta, R., Gilles, H. M. and Sandosham, A. A. (1976). Malaria in South-east Asia. *South-east Asian J. Trop. Med. Publ. Health*, **4**, 641
86. Hall, A. P. *et al.* (1977). Sequential treatment with quinine and mefloquine or quinine and pyrimethamine-sulfadoxine for falciparum malaria. *Br. Med. J.*, **1**, 1626
87. Raadt, R. de. (1976). African sleeping sickness today. *Trans. R. Soc. Trop. Med. Hyg.*, **70**, 114
88. Voller, A. (1977). Serological methods in the diagnosis of Chagas' Disease. *Trans. R. Soc. Trop. Med. Hyg.*, **71**, 10
89. Pan-American Health Organization. Scientific Publication No. 318. New approaches in American trypanosomiasis research. (Proceedings of an international symposium, Belo Horizonte, Minas Gerais, Brazil, 18–21 March 1975)
90. Jeffrey, G. M. (1958). Epidemiologic considerations of isosporiasis in a school for mental defectives. *Am. J. Hyg.* **67**, 241
91. Campos, R., Amato, N. V. and Lacerda, C. L. (1969). Brote de isosporisis en niños de un orfelinato. *Boletin Chileno de Parasitologia*, **24**, 127
92. Webster, B. A. (1957). Human isosporiasis: a report of three cases with necropsy findings in one case. *Am. J. Trop. Med. Hyg.*, **6**, 86
93. Jarpa Gana, A. (1966). Coccidiosis humana. *Biologia Santiago*, **39**, 3
94. Rommel, M. and Heydorn, A. O. (1972). Beitrag zum Lebenszyklus der Sarkosporidien. III. Isospora hominis (Raillet und Lucet 1891) Wenyon 1923, eir Dauerform der Sarkosporidien des Rinder unde des Schweim. *Berliner und Münchener Teierarztliche Wochenschrift*, **85**, 143
95. Arean, V. M. and Koppisch, E. (1956). Balantidiasis. A review and report of cases. *Am. J. Pathol.*, **32**, 1089
96. Delgado y Garnica, R., Brito Lugo, P. and Clark y Rodriguez Leal, R. (1971). Balantidiasis en la Ciudad de Mexico. *Revista Investigacion en Salud Publica*, **31**, 106
97. Garnham, P. C. C. *et al.* (1969). Human Babesiosis in Ireland: Further observations and the medical significance of this infection. *Br. Med. J.*, **4**, 768

8
Man and His Pets

D. E. JACOBS

INTRODUCTION

Some 9000 years ago, man started to impose his will on the lifestyle of wild animals and the long process of domestication commenced. The species he chose were to provide food and manure, clothing and leather, transport and power, employment and protection, company and recreation. In return man catered for the basic biological needs of his adopted creatures, although often in an inept, negligent or cruel fashion. In recent years the concept of animal welfare has evolved and is now widely practised in the western world. Thus over the centuries a mutual dependence has arisen between man and the domesticated animals. Particularly close associations have developed with the horse, dog and cat as all of these are capable of responding to affection and are often kept purely for the sake of companionship. Being of an exploratory nature, man is constantly attempting to extend the range of species that will fulfil this role: small mammals, birds, fish, reptiles and even more exotic forms of life have been subjected to captivity in his home. So close is the association between man and his animals that the pet is frequently an important component of the domestic environment. Indeed, as traditional family structures are eroded by the demands of modern society, pets are proving to be of increasing value for the psychological welfare of Western man[1].

In 1973, 33.4 million dogs and 33.6 million cats were shared amongst 38% and 23% of American households respectively[2]. There were also at that time 7 million horses in the USA, while in western Europe there were 29 million dogs, 26 million cats and 20 million cage birds. The highest concentration of dogs was found to be in Belgium with 33 per sq km but at the other end of the spectrum only 9% of families in western Germany kept dogs and only 7% owned cats.

Not every activity of the pet animal is advantageous to man. For example, unrestrained animals can cause accidents and injury, while the indiscriminate deposition of excreta can create a pollution problem. Just as man suffers from numerous diseases, so too do his companion animals. Many of these diseases are species-specific but some may be transmitted to man (zoonoses). Conversely, the pet may fall victim to some diseases of man (anthroponoses), although many infections, e.g. *Enterobius*, are restricted in their host range and cannot become established in non-primates. Additionally, there are instances where man and his pets are susceptible to the same disease without there being any risk of cross-infection. Thus a dog or cat that has consumed undercooked trichinous meat presents no danger to man, or *vice versa*.

The clinical effects of zoonotic disease range from aesthetic repugnance to death. Some infections of animal origin, however, may be beneficial if the organism is innocuous to man but capable of evoking an immunity to related pathogens (zooprophylaxis).

If the detrimental aspects of a particular form of pet ownership are unacceptable to society, remedial action must be taken. Before limiting man's freedom to possess pets, however, it is essential that public opinion should be based on a realistic appraisal of scientific fact weighing alleged offences against the benefits of pet ownership. The following pages summarize the information currently available on one important aspect of these considerations: parasitic diseases transmissible from animals to man.

The parasites of pet animals that infect man may be conveniently divided into those that are regularly transmitted via environmental contamination or by close physical contact and those that apparently invade the human body only rarely. In this chapter the term 'pet' has been interpreted as including 'companion' animals.

TRANSMISSION VIA THE ENVIRONMENT

The three parasites in this category utilize man as an integral part of their life cycle. They are all parasites of carnivores that employ a wide variety of potential prey animals as intermediate or paratenic hosts. The flesh of man is unlikely to be eaten by his pet animals, but at an earlier stage of our evolution our predecessors could well have fallen victim to the ancestors of today's canine or feline hosts, thereby enabling the parasite to complete its life cycle. 'The wolf, disarmed of ferocity, is now pillowed in the lady's lap. The cat, the little tiger of our island, whose natural home is the forest, is equally domesticated and caressed'[3].

Echinococcus

Echinococcus granulosus is a tapeworm of dogs and other Canidae that grows to a length of just a few millimetres. Yet despite the diminutive size of the adult worm, the intermediate form in man, the hydatid cyst, can grow to the size of a football. The consequences of this space-occupying lesion have been discussed in Chapter 6.

Figure 8.1   Life cycle of the strains of *Echinococcus granulosus* found in Great Britain

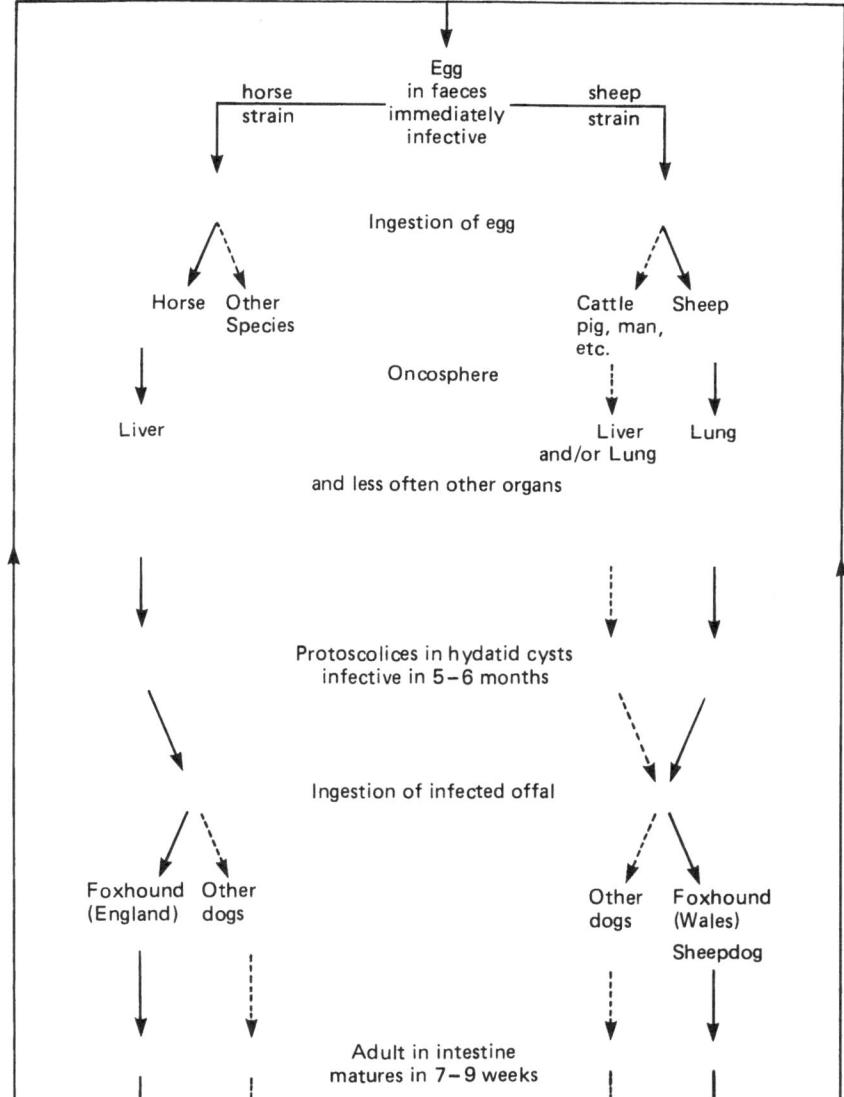

The life cycle of *E. granulosus* is displayed in Figure 8.1. This cestode can utilize a wide variety of mammalian intermediate hosts but ecological factors determine the range of potential recipient species in any geographical location or period of evolutionary history. By adapting to such situations, *E. granulosus* has split into subspecies and strains which vary in biological characteristics. This is of practical significance as different strains are often of greater or lesser infectivity for man. Also, host specificity has an important influence on the epidemiology of hydatid disease in any district. Thus, reindeer–dog and moose–wolf cycles occur in the endemic area of north-western Canada and Alaska, while a wallaby–dingo cycle is seen in Australia. It is, however, the sheep–dog cycle which is of greatest importance in most areas of the temperate world where hydatid disease of man is a problem i.e. New Zealand, New South Wales, Tasmania, the south-western United States and parts of Argentina, Uruguay and the British Isles. Man himself is often to blame when transmission occurs in lowland areas where sheep are kept intensively. This is because the life cycle is mostly perpetuated by the feeding of infected offal from slaughtered animals to working or pet dogs. The cycle can also flourish where sheep are grazed extensively in difficult upland terrain. Under these circumstances, sheepdogs find and scavenge the carcasses of animals that succumb to the harsh conditions, while the sheep in turn are exposed to high concentrations of *E. granulosus* eggs when they are gathered onto land near the farm buildings for lambing, dipping, etc.[4] These, however, are agricultural situations and so further discussion of the dog–sheep cycle and the control of hydatid disease is deferred until the final chapter of this book.

There is one epidemiological cycle that is totally confined to companion animals—the dog and the horse—which is particularly prevalent in the British Isles. During the period 1970–74, 21 people died from hydatidosis in England and 11 in Wales, but this is the tip of the iceberg. For example, the annual incidence in Powys (mid-Wales) has been estimated at 4–5 per 10 000, while 15 of 147 volunteers in this district gave positive reactions to an indirect haemagglutination test[5]. The geographical distribution of these cases, which are largely confined to Wales, the north-west of England and London, suggests man's involvement in the sheep–dog cycle in provincial areas and the importation of infections acquired overseas in the metropolis. Even, so, the occurrence of the horse strain, *E. granulosus equinus*, is causing anxiety at the present time as the prevalence in horses has risen steeply in recent years from under 10% to between 35 and 60%[6]. Studies in laboratory animals show that the cystic forms of the equine strain grow more slowly than those of the sheep strain. It has been surmised, therefore, that if the increased incidence in the horse is reflected by a similar trend in man, a number of years will elapse before the infections become clinically apparent. Fortunately, there is circumstantial evidence suggesting that this concern is misdirected. In Ireland, where the horse strain is common and yet the sheep cycle is non-existent, human cases of hydatidosis are rarely recorded. Additionally, attempts to infect non-human primates with *E. granulosus equinus* have so far been unsuccessful. The main source of infection for horses appears to be the hunting dog, while the reason for the increasing prevalence of this condition is attributed to the fact that raw horse meat and offal constitute a larger part of the diet of hounds than formerly.

Echinococcus multilocularis

Echinococcus multilocularis forms a tumour-like structure in the liver which gives the appearance of a malignant growth. There was much argument in the past as to whether the alveolar type of cyst was a special form of *E. granulosus* cyst or a separate species. It is now firmly established that *E. granulosus* does not produce the multilocular or alveolar cyst which is the intermediate stage of *E. multilocularis*. The definitive hosts are dogs, foxes and cats. The intermediate hosts are microtine rodents and it is propagated in a sylvatic cycle through foxes and mice. As cats more frequently consume mice than do dogs, cats are more likely to be a source of infection for man than dogs.

As this parasite has only recently been recognized as different from *E. granulosus* its distribution is not well documented. In the USSR *E. multilocularis* has a relatively wide distribution in foxes and man[7]. Up to 70% of foxes in Siberia have been reported to be infected. In North America it is chiefly confined to the islands off Alaska and some infection occurs on the adjacent mainland but not elsewhere on the American continent. In Europe there are records of its occurrence in Germany and Switzerland.

Control is difficult since it is almost impossible to break the sylvatic cycle. Steps should be taken to eliminate tapeworms from cats and also dogs in order to reduce the chances of infection of man. The control of mice can assist in reducing the chances of domestic cats becoming infected.

Toxocara

The second member of the trio of genera exploiting predator–prey relationships is a nematode, *Toxocara*, which exists as two separate species: *T. canis* and *T. cati*, the adults of which are found in the small intestine of the dog and cat respectively. Larval forms of each species invade the tissues of a wide spectrum of vertebrates, including man (Figure 8.3). A third ascarid species, *Toxascaris leonina*, parasitizes cats and dogs and although it too utilizes potential prey animals in its life cycle, human infections have not so far been recognized. All these parasites are similar in appearance but patent infections in cats or dogs can be differentiated without difficulty as the eggs of *Toxocara* spp. are brown with a pitted shell, whereas *Toxascaris* ova are smooth and colourless (Figure 8.2). The adult worms can grow to a length of 18 cm and are occasionally found in the intestines of man[8] but more often it is the larvae that occur in human tissues. These are rather less than half a millimetre long. Identification of the larvae in histological sections is a highly skilled procedure described by Nichols[9].

The life cycles of the two *Toxocara* species differ markedly and each involves several routes of transmission. The key to the epidemiology of toxocariasis is the egg contaminating the environment and so this is the most appropriate point to commence the description of the complex life cycle of this

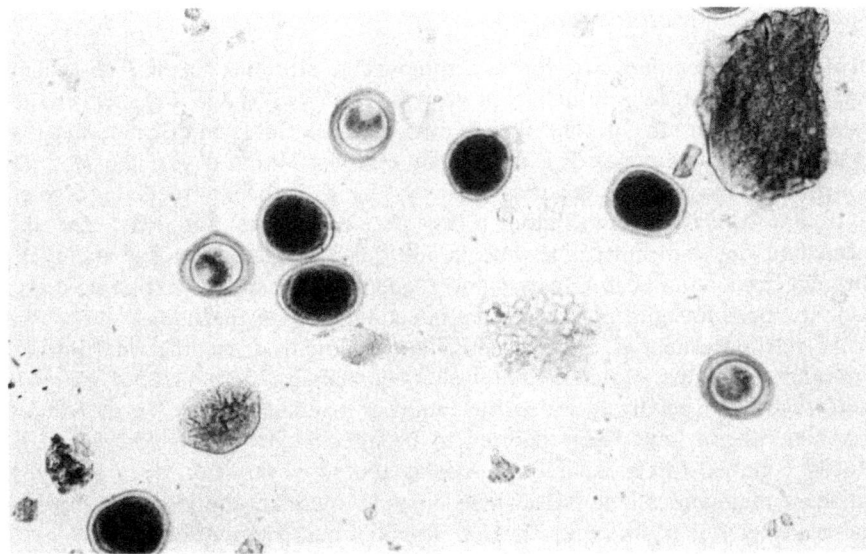

Figure 8.2 *Toxocara canis* eggs (dark) and *Toxascaris leonina* ova (pale) as they appear in a fresh preparation of canine faeces (Photograph from Pegg. E. J. and Shephard, R., *Journal of Small Animal Practice,* **7**, 457. 1966)

group (Figure 8.4). When embryonated ova of *Toxocara* are ingested by a bitch or queen, the larvae hatch out, penetrate the wall of the intestine and, without growing or developing, enter a waiting phase in various tissues, including the kidneys, liver and musculature. If the bitch becomes pregnant, a proportion of the accumulated *T. canis* larvae cross the placenta making their way to the foetal liver. The remaining larvae are available as a source of infection for future litters. By the time the pups are born, many larvae will have migrated to the lungs on their way via the trachea and oesophagus to the small intestine where they will become adult. Prenatal infection does not take place in the cat. The most important mode of transmission in this species occurs after parturition when *T. cati* larvae appear in the mammary glands and pass into the suckling kittens with the milk. Galactogenic infection also occurs with *T. canis* but this is of secondary importance. Larvae from embryonated eggs ingested by pups and kittens will migrate by the tracheal route to the intestine, but as the animals grow older an increasing proportion will make their way instead to the somatic tissues.

Thus the life cycle of *Toxocara*, unlike that of *Echinococcus*, can proceed without the use of potential prey animals, but if the embryonated egg in the environment is taken up by such an animal a somatic infection results. The larva is able to resume its development if the paratenic host is eaten by the appropriate predator. Hence, it is almost impossible for a cat owner to keep a

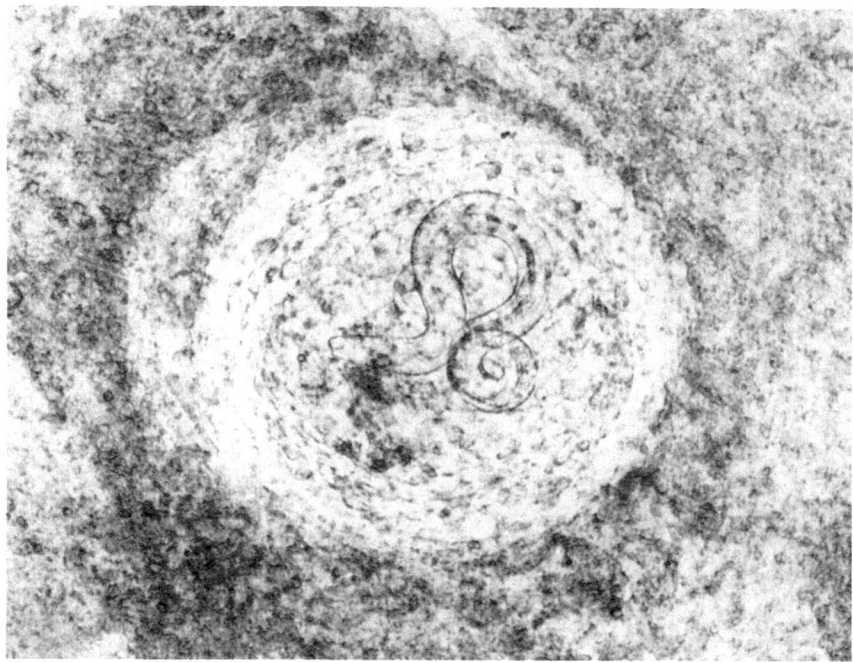

Figure 8.3 Larva of *Toxocara canis* in a granuloma (Photograph Dr G. J. Kane, Wellcome Research Laboratories)

good mouser free of worms.

Man is usually infected with *Toxocara* when he ingests embryonated ova contaminating his fingers or food, but larvae may also be acquired from eating undercooked meat derived from animals that have themselves swallowed embryonated *Toxocara* eggs. This, however, is probably a rare occurrence in western countries. In pigs, for example, the larvae are relatively short-lived and only 0.06% were found to have high antibody titres to this parasite in Britain[10].

The term *visceral larva migrans* has been used to refer to the passage of larvae through the human body[11,12]. In the United Kingdom, between 2 and 5% of the adult population give positive reactions to immunodiagnostic tests used by the Toxocaral Reference Laboratory in London[13]. Higher prevalences are, however, found in certain groups of patients such as those with choroidoretinitis, hepatomegaly with eosinophilia, idiopathic asthma, poliomyelitis and epilepsy, suggesting either a greater exposure to infection or the involvement of the parasite in the disease process. This can be the result of massive larval invasion or the chance occurrence of a larva in a critical tissue (such as the retina), or possibly of indirect effects such as the production of an

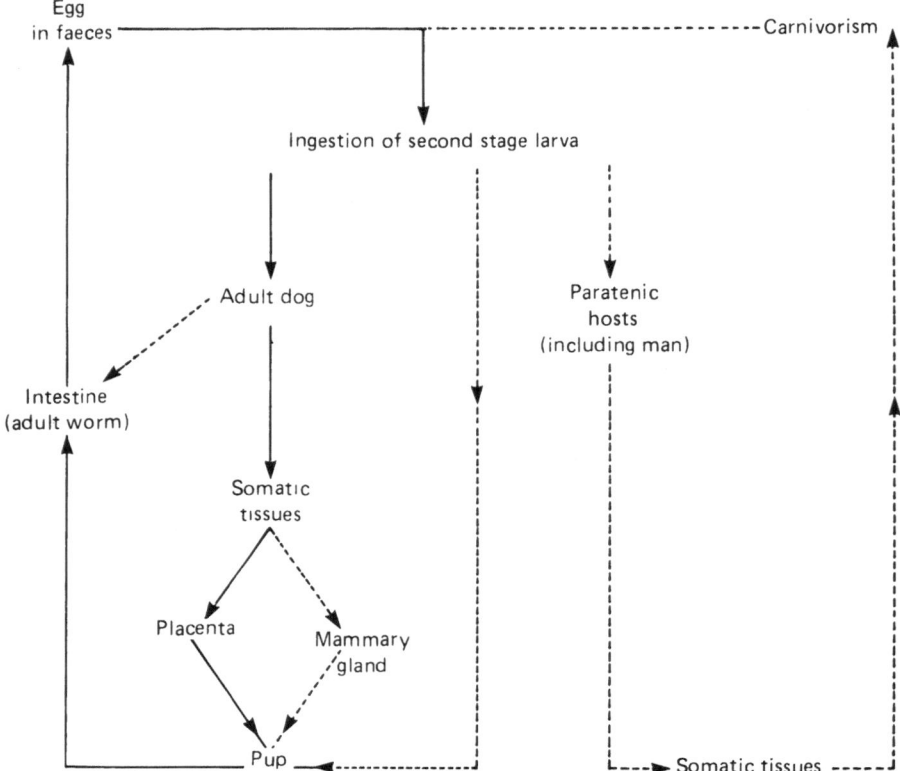

Figure 8.4   Life cycle of *Toxocara canis*

allergic response or the exacerbation of a pre-existing condition. Children are particularly at risk since they are more likely to ingest contaminated soil or faeces. It is difficult to quantify the extent of human suffering caused by *Toxocara*, but in Great Britain, with a population of some 55 millions, 54 cases with ocular involvement were recorded by the Toxocaral Reference Laboratory during 1977[14].

The acquisition of large numbers of larvae will produce a generalized syndrome with eosinophilia, pyrexia and hepatomegaly, sometimes accompanied by encephalitis, dyspnoea or a skin reaction, often associated with a history of pica (Chapter 5). Such cases are fortunately rare in the United Kingdom but occur more frequently in socially disadvantaged communities living in warmer, wetter climates. Under such conditions, *Toxocara* eggs, which are not immediately infective when passed in the faeces of the canine or feline host, are likely to accumulate and embryonate quickly. In more temperate areas, development of the ova is restricted to the summer months. During the maturation period the faeces may be dispersed and the eggs disseminated by natural forces such as wind and rain. Thus there is little correlation between the occurrence of ova in gardens, or antibodies to *Toxocara* in children, and pet ownership. Many eggs probably have a short lifespan but some can remain viable for at least two years.

Surveys in Europe and North America have revealed a substantial reservoir of infection in the urban environment[15,16]. Between 5 and 25% of soil samples taken from gardens, parks, sandpits, etc., have been shown to contain *Toxocara* eggs. As might be expected, ova are more abundant in large kennel establishments but only a proportion will be embryonated at any one time (fewer than 1% during a British winter, for example). Investigations in the United Kingdom suggest that infection with *T. canis* is acquired only infrequently by knowledgeable dog handlers[17]. Thus at greyhound kennels where 500 racing dogs were shedding 19 million *Toxocara* ova daily onto a 56 hectare estate, only two long-term employees from a total of 34 kennel workers were shown to possess demonstrable antibodies.

The eggs in the urban environment originate from the faeces of dogs, foxes or cats but unfortunately there is no practical means of differentiating ova from these three sources. In Europe, red foxes frequently harbour *T. canis* and are known to inhabit some urban areas, but population densities are probably not great enough to contaminate their surroundings to a significant extent. In many localities, up to 35% of cats shed *T. cati* ova and this animal may be responsible for some cases of clinical or asymptomatic *Toxocara* infections in man, but its importance in this respect is largely speculative at the present time.

The prevalence of *T. canis* in dogs varies from 2 to 60% in Europe, North America and Australia, depending on the source and type of animal and the age and sex distribution of the sample. In the UK, for example, the average infestation rate is in the region of 11 to 13% with lower values recorded for pampered pets and figures slightly higher for large kennel establishments and much higher for some groups of city dog[15]. A very high proportion of pups are born with the infection but most of the worms are expelled during the first months of life so that the number of dogs shedding eggs declines with age. Adult male dogs are more likely to harbour egg-laying worms than are bitches.

The complex life cycle of *Toxocara* makes control of the parasite difficult even for the professional cat or dog breeder. At the time of writing, there is no anthelminthic that will kill somatic larvae in the bitch or queen, or migrating *Toxocara* larvae in the pup or kitten. The only stages in the life cycle that are susceptible to chemotherapeutic attack are the intestinal forms. Frequent anthelminthic treatments are required to prevent egg excretion by the newborn animal since new intestinal populations are quickly established following each dose. As the animal approaches adulthood, fewer treatments are required but regular worming should be accepted as an essential part of responsible pet ownership. In this way, much can be done to reduce the numbers of *Toxocara* eggs in the environment, although there will always be the problem of the fox, the neglected dog, the stray and the independent cat.

The long-lived *Toxocara* egg has a sticky coat which also serves to protect the larva within from the effects of disinfectants. The total elimination of eggs from contaminated premises can only be achieved by extreme measures such as the use of a horticultural flame gun, but as this approach is often impracticable, vigorous scrubbing with copious volumes of hot water is a good compromise. Personal hygiene is an obvious safeguard against fortuitous ingestion of ova but is difficult to impose in the case of children.

Toxoplasma

One of the most exciting parasitological events of recent years was the discovery that the potentially pathogenic tissue-dwelling protozoan *Toxoplasma gondii* is the intermediate stage of a coccidian parasite of the cat. The realization that coccidia do not always have direct life cycles but sometimes utilize intermediate hosts led immediately to an explosion of knowledge in this field of protozoology[18,19]. It was soon found that *Sarcocystis* spp. were also intermediate stages in the life cycles of similar parasites of meat-eating animals. Several new genera and many new parasitic species have been erected to accommodate the full range of forms that have since been described and new information on their life cycles is emerging month by month. At the time of writing, however, the only parasite of this group that is known to be transmitted from companion animals to man is *Toxoplasma*.

The relationship between *T. gondii* and its non-definitive hosts, which include almost all warm-blooded vertebrates, is more complex than is the case with the two helminth parasites decribed earlier in this section. One ingested egg of *Toxocara*, for example, can give rise to only one somatic larva. Similarly, an *Echinococcus* egg typically produces a single hydatid cyst but this contains thousands of infective protoscolices. *Toxoplasma* takes this sequence one step further—not only is asexual multiplication a feature of this part of the life cycle but horizontal and vertical transmission can take place within the intermediate host population. Thus, one toxoplasmal oocyst has the potential to produce countless infective cysts in innumerable potential prey animals. The life cycle is completed if the flesh of one of these is eaten by a cat or certain other felidae (Figure 8.5).

Two main forms of the parasite occur in the intermediate host. In the acute phase of the infection, the predominant form is the tachyzoite, which is roughly banana-shaped and about 6 μm long. Dissemination through the body may take place by local migration, passage across serous cavities, transport within mobile host cells or via the lymphatics and blood. Associated pathological changes have been described in Chapter 7. If parasitaemia coincides with pregnancy, the organism may invade the tissues of the foetus, although the

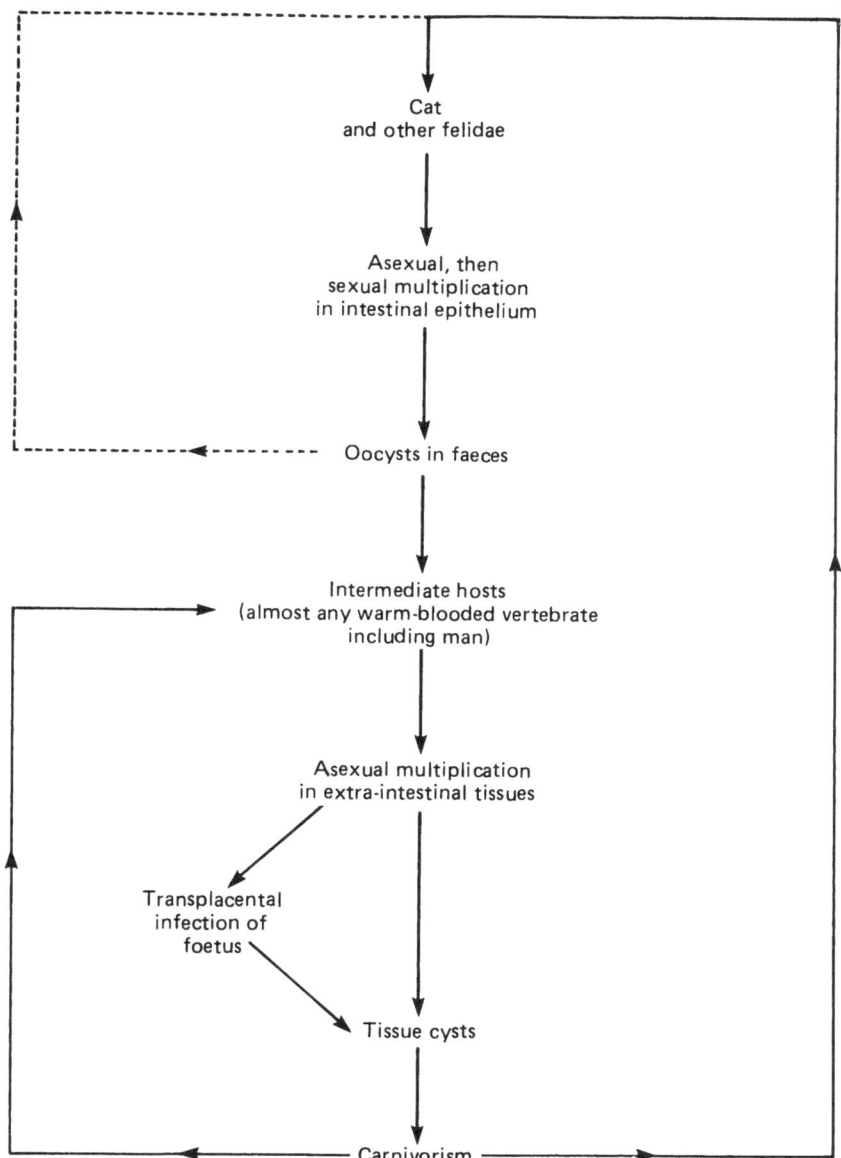

Figure 8.5   Life cycle of *Toxoplasma gondii*

mechanism involved and the consequences vary with factors such as the type of placentation of the host species. In the mouse, a single experimental infection of a gravid female may lead to the infection being passed through ten subsequent generations[20].

On entering a host cell, the tachyzoite reproduces rapidly and the resulting intracellular clone is known as a terminal colony or pseudocyst. When the infection passes into the chronic phase, the predominant form of the parasite is known as the bradyzoite. This divides slowly within a well-defined parasitic membrane forming the so-called tissue cyst. Transition from the acute to chronic phase occurs after a variable period which may, perhaps, be determined by host factors such as immunological responses. Toxoplasmal cysts may persist for protracted periods, particularly in nervous tissue, but the infection can revert to the acute form if the intermediate host is subjected to stress, concurrent disease or induced immunosuppression.

The definitive host, the cat, acquires infection by ingesting tachyzoites or bradyzoites in the tissues of captured rodents and birds or in contaminated uncooked meat. The sporulated oocyst is of low infectivity when swallowed by the cat. In place of the schizogony of conventional coccidia, *Toxoplasma* invades the epithelial cells of the small intestine and undergoes a complex process of asexual replication involving numerous generations and five distinct morphological types. Gametogony takes place between the third and 15th days after infection during which time over a billion oocysts are discharged into the intestinal contents. The oocysts of *T. gondii* are much smaller than those of the feline *Isospora* spp. (now known as *Cystoisospora* or *Levineia* spp.) measuring 10 × 12 μm (Figure 8.6). After sporulation, each oocyst contains two sporocysts each with four sporozoites. For a certain diagnosis, however, it is necessary to inoculate mice with faecal material as it is impossible to distinguish morphologically between the oocysts of *T. gondii* and those of a related organism, *Hammondia hammondi*[19]. The latter has not as yet been implicated in human disease. Toxoplasmal oocysts, like the ova of *Toxocara*, are extremely resistant to most external influences and may retain their infectivity for prolonged periods. They can be disseminated mechanically by invertebrates as well as by natural forces.

The sexual cycle in the intestine is self-limiting and the cat is subsequently not susceptible to reinfection, although patent infections can recur should immunity wane. Up to two-thirds of a cat population may be seropositive to *T. gondii*, but only about 1% are likely to be shedding oocysts at any one time. Epidemiological studies in Kansas City suggest that hunting is an important factor in the transmission of the parasite[21]. Infection was more common in stray cats (57.9%) than domestic cats (37.5%), while much lower prevalences were demonstrated in pet animals under six months of age. Transplacental infection does not take place in this species.

It is not known to what extent human infection is attributable, directly or indirectly, to contamination of the environment by oocysts of feline origin. The inhabitants of remote islands devoid of cats are, however, almost invariably seronegative suggesting that the presence of the definitive host is essential for the maintenance of the life cycle[22]. Nevertheless, it is generally considered that transmission to man commonly occurs as a result of handling or eating raw or undercooked meat (particularly rabbit, pork and mutton) containing

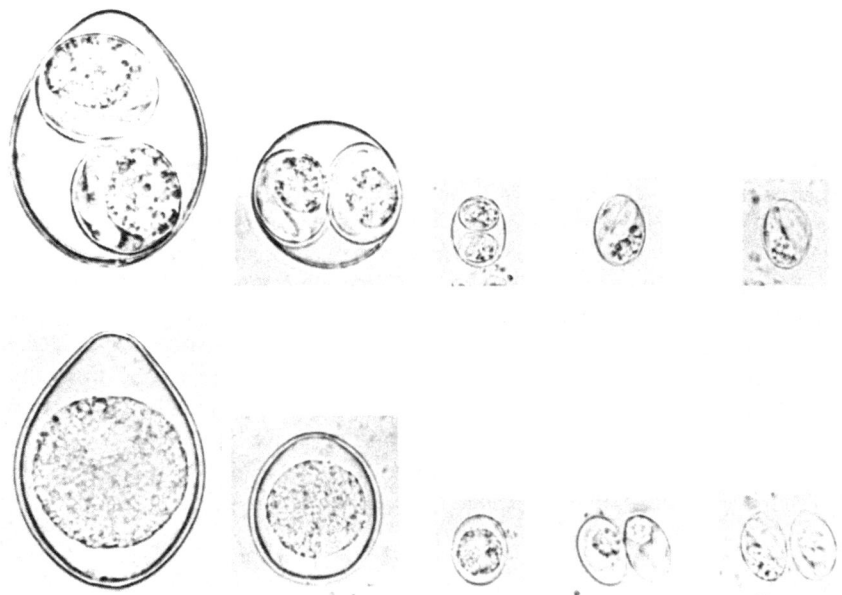

Figure 8.6 Coccidial oocysts and sporocysts from the faeces of the cat. From left to right: *Cystoisospora felis; C. rivolta; Toxoplasma gondii: Sarcocystis ovifelis* and *S. bovifelis.* To scale: the oocyst of *T. gondii* measures approximately 12 × 10 μm. (Photograph from Rommel M., *Berliner und Münchener tierärtzliche Wochenschrift,* **88,** 112. 1975)

toxoplasmal cysts or pseudocysts (Chapter 7). Adequate cooking of meat and kitchen hygiene will obviously reduce this risk, but prophylactic measures must also take account of infection via the oocyst.

Unfortunately, efforts to reduce the numbers of oocysts entering the environment are likely to have no more than a marginal effect. Domestic cats that eat nothing but canned food or cooked meat are unlikely to become infected but will fail to develop an immunity. A spirited cat, however, will supplement its ration by its own ingenuity thereby exposing itself to infection. The period of patency is transient and its onset unpredictable, so that suppression by chemotherapy is rarely practicable. This is especially true of the independent animal. A more rational approach would be vaccination but a great deal of research is required before this objective can be attained[23]. Meanwhile, litter-trays should be cleaned daily so that the excreta can be destroyed before the oocysts sporulate. Little can be done to prevent the contamination of garden soil but children's sand-boxes should be covered when not in use. As with *Toxocara* and *Echinococcus,* application of the elementary rules of hygiene will reduce the risk of ingesting infective material.

TRANSMISSION VIA CLOSE CONTACT WITH PETS

The parasites so far discussed have been characterized by the widespread dissemination of their eggs or oocysts in the environment. In contrast, the epidemiological feature shared by the next series of organisms, all ectoparasites, is that transmission is unlikely to occur unless the human sufferer is in continual physical contact with an infected pet animal or, in some cases, the animal's habitual haunts. Members of this group are commonly associated with skin disease in man. In one rural area of England, for example, more than 5% of patients entering dermatology clinics had complaints directly attributable to animal ectoparasites[24]. It is also true that pets are sometimes put down as a consequence of mistaken suspicion of zoonotic involvement. Care is therefore required with diagnosis to avoid unnecessary grief and destruction.

The life cycles and biology of the different types of ectoparasite that live on man have been described in Chapters 2–4 and need not be repeated here. The following paragraphs will be restricted to an account of zoonotic relationships concerning fleas, ticks, mites and lice.

Fleas

Few cats and dogs in any part of the world pass through life without becoming at least temporarily infested with fleas (Figure 8.7). This applies to pampered

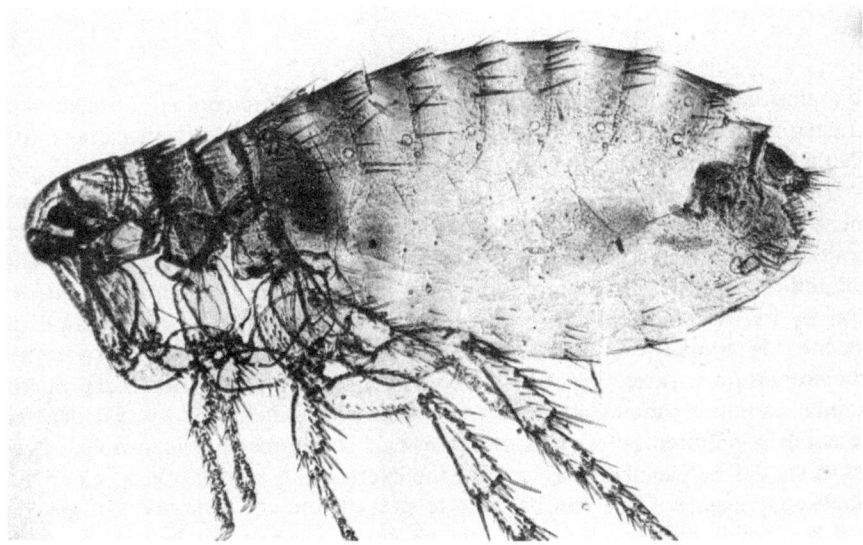

Figure 8.7   The dog flea, *Ctenocephalides canis*. (Photograph from Pegg, E. J. and Shephard, R., *Journal of Small Animal Practice*, **7**, 457. 1966)

pets as well as the less well-cared-for, although the latter often support a more abundant population. In a survey conducted recently in London, 16.9% of 136 dogs and 58.3% of 127 cats harboured fleas[25]. Such infestations often pass unnoticed. In one American study, for example, 279 of 416 affected dogs showed no clinical evidence of their ectoparasitic fauna[26].

The spectrum of flea species on pets varies with the geographical locality and special groups of animals may possess a characteristic fauna. For example, the most common flea on English dogs is the cat flea, *Ctenocephalides felis felis*, while the dog flea, *Ctenocephalides canis*, is relatively uncommon except in racing greyhounds where it is the dominant species. Greyhounds sometimes harbour the human flea, *Pulex irritans*, which otherwise is virtually non-existent in Great Britain[25]. In the neighbouring country of Ireland, on the other hand, 86% of a series of 50 dogs carried *C. canis*, 24% *P. irritans* and only 4% *C. felis*[27]. The dog flea does not seem to be able to survive on feline hosts as very few were found on cats in the English investigation, but other species found on pets included the rabbit flea (*Spilopsyllus cuniculi*), the hedgehog flea (*Archaeopsyllus erinacei erinacei*) and the bird flea (*Ceratophyllus gallinae*). Additionally, European and Oriental rat fleas and sticktight fleas have been recovered from dogs in Australia.

The demise of *P. irritans* in developed countries is attributed to changes in the domestic habitat associated with the style of modern living. However, the conditions inimical to *Pulex* seem ideal for *C. felis* which can breed freely in many homes, offices and even hospitals. Unsuspected infections on pets, or infestation on unsuspected commensal stray cats, can supply a constant source of flea eggs. These can develop almost undisturbed in the pile of fitted carpets, behind wall panelling, in air ducting or perhaps in the pet's basket or favourite armchair (Figure 8.8). Problems are particularly severe in warmer areas such as the south-eastern United States or during hot summer periods in more temperate areas. A tenfold increase in the number of enquiries regarding cat and dog fleas was recorded between 1969 and 1975 by the Danish State Pest Laboratory[28].

Cat, dog and bird fleas, together with those of several wild animals, are all capable of feeding on man, mostly evoking pleomorphic papular urticarial reactions varying in severity from individual to individual[24]. Continued exposure may result in a loss of skin reactivity to flea bites.

Hungry fleas are acquired from places frequented by the carrier animal rather than from the reservoir host itself. Thus the first bites usually occur on the ankles of the victim, who need not necessarily be the owner of the offending pet. To control flea infestations, therefore, it is necessary to trace the source of the problem and then destroy the eggs, larvae, pupae and imago fleas in the companion animal's surroundings. Otherwise the pet will quickly become reinfested after each insecticidal treatment, and the risk to humans will continue. Pupae can remain viable for months, especially if the house is left empty. The fleas will then become active when the building is reoccupied. As pets can

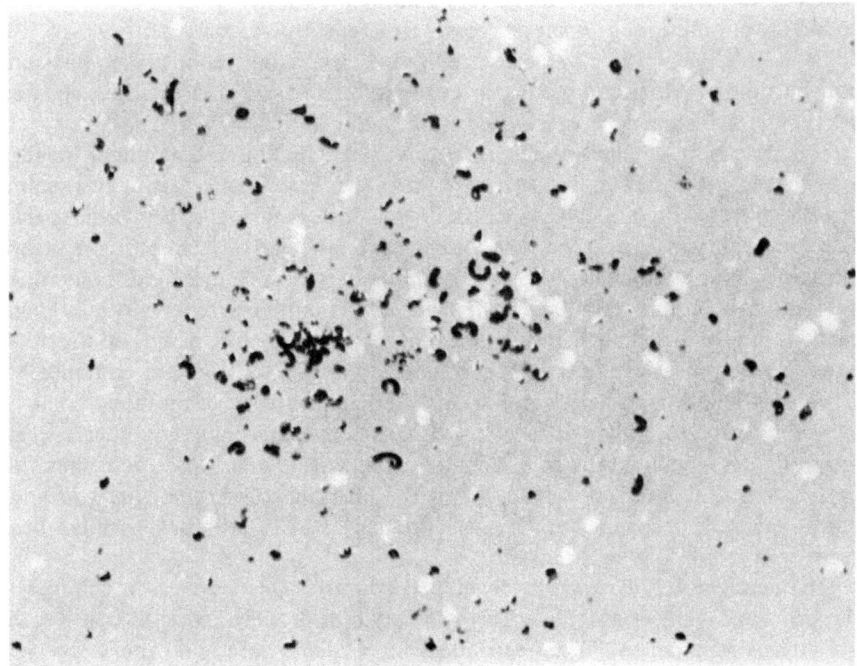

Figure 8.8 'Flea dirt'—flea eggs and excreta that have fallen from an animal carrying the adult parasite. (Photograph Mr L. R. Thomsett)

so easily acquire new infestations in both urban and rural environments, prophylactic collars have been manufactured that emit a constant flow of insecticide into the animal's coat.

Ticks

Most ticks recovered from cats, dogs and man in Europe have a wide host range and almost invariably the primary sources of infection are either farm livestock or wild animals. Examples are *Ixodes ricinus* (the sheep tick), *Ixodes hexagonus* (the hedgehog tick) and *Dermacentor reticulatus*, which is common in France. In Australia, *Ixodes holocyclus*, a parasite of the bandicoot, can cause paralysis in dogs and man. Specific dog ticks do occur, however, such as *Ixodes canisuga,* found on greyhounds in Britain. Of greater importance is *Dermacentor variabilis* (the American dog tick) which is widespread in the eastern United States and Canada. It is not uncommon for humans fondling infested dogs to acquire these ticks which are capable of transmitting Rocky Mountain Spotted Fever and producing tick paralysis. The brown dog tick, *Rhipicephalus sanguineus*, is of veterinary interest as the vector of canine piroplasmosis. It is of particular nuisance value to man as, like the cat flea, it thrives in the modern home and is partial to human blood. It is of almost cosmopolitan distribution but is absent from northern Europe and some parts of Canada. Serious problems have arisen, however, in centrally heated homes in the latter areas following the importation of dogs from endemic zones[29]. Eradication is difficult and involves the application of acaricides to the hiding places of the non-parasitic forms as well as the treatment of the animal. In Scandinavia, the most effective cure is for the suffering family to take a winter holiday, leaving their home without heating for a sufficient period of time to kill the ticks.

Exotic pets, especially from tropical areas, may be accompanied by an interesting variety of ectoparasites. Nasty bites can be inflicted, for example, by ixodid ticks (*Hyalomma* spp.) from tortoises.

Mites

The acari of zoonotic importance present a wide range of parasitic relationships and cognisance of these is necessary for an understanding of the epidemiology of each condition and associated control strategies. At one end of the spectrum, the ovigerous females of *Sarcoptes scabiei* var. *canis* and its feline counterpart *Notoedres cati* are in intimate contact with host tissue, spending the greater part of their lives in skin burrows. *Cheyletiella* spp. are also permanent parasites but all stages are 'free-living' on the surface of the skin. *Dermanyssus gallinae*, the red mite of poultry and other birds, inhabits buildings and attaches to its host only when it requires a blood meal. The harvest mites are also transient parasites but they live outdoors showing little host preference.

Evidence is accruing that animal scabies is highly contagious to man. Notoedric mange is very rare in domestic cats but sarcoptic mange, for example, was diagnosed in 0.71% of 56 394 dogs seen at a clinic in Scotland[30]. Extrapolation of this figure suggests that there may be in excess of 40 000 infected dogs in the United Kingdom, each exposing its owner and his family, neighbours and visitors to risk. In an investigation of 65 people in contact with 42 mite-infested pets (28 harbouring *Sarcoptes* and the remainder *Cheyletiella*), 50 showed lesions of acariasis, 34 of which were due to canine scabies[31].

The lesions in man differ from those of human scabies in appearance and distribution. The mite is capable of migrating through clothing but will not form burrows in human skin. Reactions range from an irritant papular rash to a severe sensitivity response and are confined to those areas of the body that come into apposition with the carrier animal, e.g. the forearms, the lap, etc. As the association of this mite with man is transient and superficial, confirmation of diagnosis is dependent upon the veterinary examination of contact animals. The demonstration of the causal organism in dogs can, however, be difficult and if direct microscopical examination of deep skin scrapings treated with 10% KOH is unsuccessful, concentration techniques must be used. Remission of symptoms in the human patient will only be possible if the source of infection is removed, either by curing the animal or, in intransigent cases, by euthanasia.

Similar mites parasitizing rodents, birds and exotic species have been reported occasionally as the cause of dermatitis in man. Quite different circumstances pertain with mites such as *Dermanyssus* as no direct contact with the infected animals is necessary for transmission to occur. In fact, the danger to man is enhanced if the natural host is absent (for example, an empty poultry house, pigeon loft or a deserted bird's nest in the eaves of a house) as there may then be a large number of unfed mites seeking a host. Obviously, the avoidance of the intense discomfort evoked in man by the Red Mite depends upon the treatment of all potential breeding sites in the affected building as well as the application of acaricides to the birds in his care.

Another mite that can cause intense irritation, but in this case in people that nurse infected animals in their arms or on their laps, is *Cheyletiella*. Not all persons at risk develop lesions but of those that do approximately one-third display small red macules that develop to form yellow crusted lesions with central necrosis[24]. The remainder may show a variety of cutaneous changes. Although the first human case was diagnosed as long ago as 1918, it is only in recent years that the true extent of human involvement has been realized. Like *Sarcoptes*, this mite is a transient visitor unable to establish itself on man. The difficulties of diagnosis are compounded by the fact that the source of infection may remain unsuspected as the signs of *Cheyletiella* infestation in animals are often confined to a slight tendency to dandruff and hyperaesthesia of the skin. Infestation can be demonstrated by rigorous grooming of the animal over a large sheet of paper. The highly motile mites can just be seen with the naked eye in the brushings but positive identification requires microscopic confirmation of the presence of powerful claws on the palps (Figure 8.9).

There are five known species of *Cheyletiella* on pet animals: *C. parasitivorax* and two others on rabbits, *C. yasguri* on dogs (Figure 8.10) and *C. blakei* on cats. Species identification is extremely complex and in consequence literature references to the epidemiology of *Cheyletiella* infections are confused by the possibility of misidentification[32]. However, it is suspected that *C. parasitivorax* and *C. yasguri* at least can complete their life cycle only on their natural hosts, infestations on other hosts being short-lived and abortive. The lesions on man will regress spontaneously soon after the elimination of the animal infection.

The last group of mites are not specifically parasites of companion animals since they readily infest a wide range of hosts including man. The only blame that can be attached to the pet in this context is that it may be responsible for acquiring the organisms in rough undergrowth and transferring them to the domestic environment. Included in this category are the harvest mite (*Trom-*

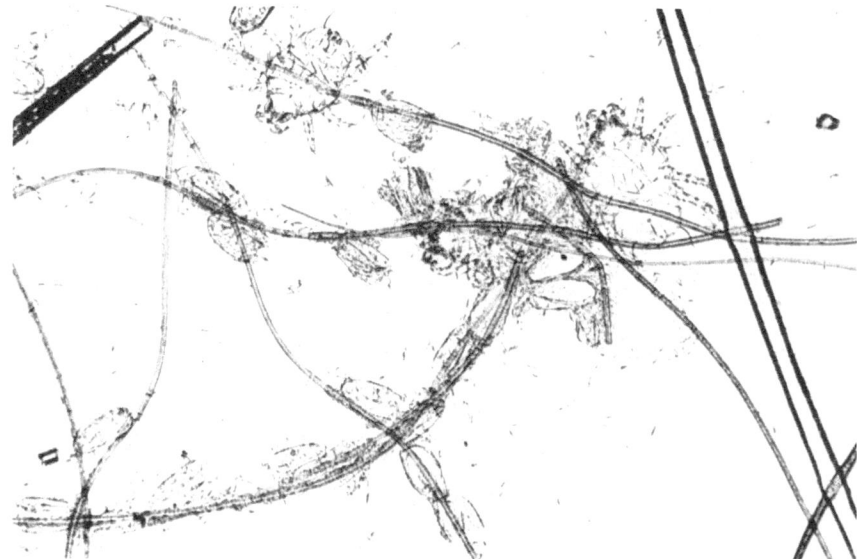

Figure 8.9 *Cheyletiella* spp.—adults and eggs in animal hair. Note the strong claws on the palps. (Photograph Mr L. R. Thomsett)

bicula autumnalis) in Europe and related species in other parts of the world that enjoy names such as the scrub itch mite, velvet mite, heel bug, North American chigger, bush mokka, etc. They are all free-living organisms that require animal protein only for the development of the larval stage. The parasitic forms therefore have six legs. They usually congregate on the areas of the body with the thinnest skin, such as the interdigital spaces of dogs and the ankles, thigh, groin and waist of man.

Lice

Dogs commonly harbour both anopluran and mallophagan lice, this being particularly true of the long-haired breeds. Horses may also harbour lice of both types, while the cat is infrequently infested with sucking lice only. This group is of little zoonotic importance and should perhaps be relegated to the next section of this chapter: parasites that rarely infest man.

TRANSMISSION APPARENTLY RARE

The parasites under this heading form a miscellaneous group of little importance in general terms but they are nevertheless distressing to the few unlucky

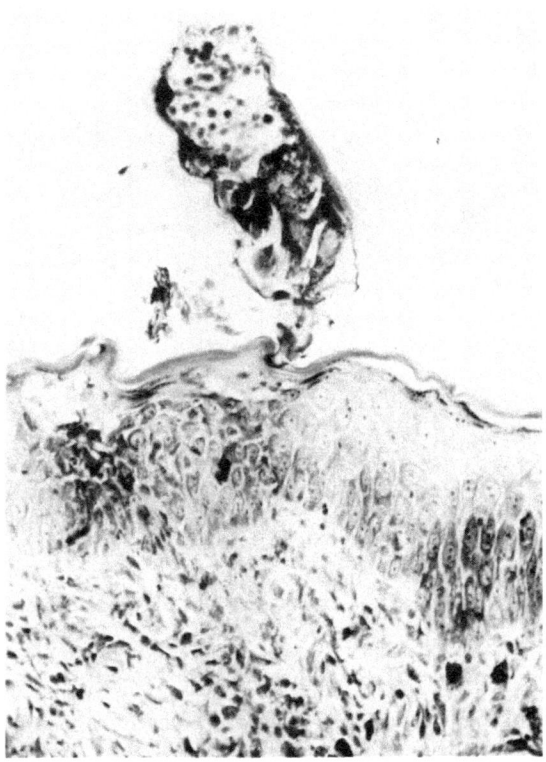

Figure 8.10   Section of *Cheyletiella* spp. biting dog skin (Photograph Mr L. R. Thomsett)

individuals whose tissues are invaded. Several different reasons may be postulated for the apparent rarity of each infection. In some cases, the parasitism is unlikely to be recognized unless the patient becomes hypersensitive (e.g. hookworm dermatitis). Alternatively, the parasite may only be detected as a result of some other diagnostic procedure (e.g. mass radiography may visualize coin lesions produced by the canine heartworm). Often infection might be more common if there were more frequent opportunities for transmission. (To acquire *Dipylidium caninum* one has to swallow an infected flea from a dog or cat, which cannot be a common occurrence!) Finally, when no other explanation is forthcoming, we may assume that the parasite is of low infectivity for man.

Taenia

At least seven species of *Taenia* occur in the dog but only two of these have so far been implicated in human disease in temperate climates. These are *T. mul-*

ticeps (syn. *Multiceps multiceps*) and *T. serialis*. Both grow up to a metre in length in the small intestine of the canine host and each has a life cycle resembling that of *T. saginata*, the beef tapeworm of man (Chapter 6). An important difference, however, is the type of metacestode that develops when the egg is ingested by the intermediate host. In place of the cysticercus (which has one inverted scolex), a shared feature of *T. multiceps* and *T. serialis* is the formation of a coenurus characterized by multiple inverted scolices. These are randomly distributed on the inner surface of the bladder wall in the former case and arranged in rows in the latter. The metacestode of *T. serialis* is typically found in the intermuscular connective tissue of rabbits while that of *T. multiceps* occurs primarily in the brain and spinal cord of sheep. The latter is common in sheep rearing areas such as the Dyfed region of mid-Wales where 11.5% of sheepdogs and 5.8% of lambs are infected[33], while *T. serialis* infections are likely to be found wherever dogs can feed on rabbit carcasses. Thus infection is largely confined to rural areas.

Cerebral infections of man are reported rarely—four times in France, twice in England and the USA, and eight times in other countries[34,35]. The symptomatology is that associated with a space occupying lesion. The prognosis is grave, only four of 12 patients surviving craniotomy. Subcutaneous coenuri, presumably *T. serialis*, have been reported three times from France.

The cat also harbours a taeniid tapeworm, *T. taeniaformis,* the metacestode of which is called *Strobilocercus fasciolaris*. This normally occurs in rodents but has been found on one occasion in the liver of man[36].

Spirometra

This is a pseudophyllidean tapeworm with a life history similar to that of *Diphyllobothrium* (Chapter 6) except that the procercoid develops in freshwater crustacea, such as *Cyclops*, and the plerocercoid in a wide range of vertebrates including amphibians, reptiles and mammals. The plerocercoid is capable of leaving the tissues of an eaten host to invade those of the predator. Thus, man can become infected as an intermediate host by ingesting the procercoid in drinking water contaminated with *Cyclops*, or as a paratenic host by eating undercooked meat (e.g. barbecued feral pig) containing the plerocercoid. The definitive hosts are the dog and cat.

The plerocercoid of *Spirometra* is known as a 'sparganum' and may grow up to several centimetres in length, coiled in a fibrous subcutaneous nodule. Infections are largely confined to the warmer parts of the regions discussed in this book, particularly Louisiana and adjoining states (where 25 of the 35 North American cases reported up to 1964 had occurred[37]) and Australia. Different species are implicated, *S. mansonoides* in the former area and *S. erinacei* in the latter.

Dipylidium

Dipylidium caninum differs from the other zoonotic cestodes so far mentioned in this chapter in that it is not the larval form that is found in man but the adult tapeworm. This can grow to a length of 75 cm in the small intestine. Human infections are diagnosed sporadically in all parts of the world, 13 such records appearing in the American literature up to 1960[38]. Most cases occur in children and are asymptomatic but some are associated with abdominal pain, failure to gain weight and anal pruritus.

The usual definitive hosts, cats and dogs, frequently harbour *D. caninum.* The motile proglottids are expelled with the faeces or leave independently through the anus, often causing embarrassment to the pet owner. This response is compounded when the owner discovers that the presence of *D. caninum* is indicative of a flea infestation in the household. For the life cycle to be completed the eggs, released from the gravid segment in packets of up to 20, have to be taken up by a flea larva. The resulting cysticercoid is infective when the adult flea emerges from its pupa to seek a blood meal but infection will only take place if the flea is swallowed.

D. caninum proglottids can be recognized as they are oval rather than rectangular and have two genital pores opening laterally, one on each side.

Rodent tapeworms

Hymenolepis diminuta is a cyclophyllidean cestode of rats, mice and wild rodents that can grow to maturity in man, being reported occasionally from children in the southern United States, southern Europe and other areas of the world. Potential intermediate hosts include flour beetles. This worm is considerably longer (3–6 cm) than the dwarf tapeworm *Hymenolepis nana* (less than 0.5 cm) which is a more serious problem in human medicine. However, it is generally thought that the rodent variety of *H. nana* is physiologically distinct and unlikely to infect man.

Hookworms

There are two genera of hookworm in dogs and cats: *Ancylostoma*, composed of tropical species (although the endemic ranges of some encroach on temperate regions) and *Uncinaria* which is adapted for much colder climates, including subarctic regions. On the eastern seaboard of Australia, the only hookworm found in Brisbane dogs is *Ancylostoma* while *Uncinaria* alone occurs in Melbourne, but the two intermingle where the two ecological zones overlap in Sydney[39].

Three species of *Ancylostoma* are known to exist in dogs, *A. caninum, A. braziliense* and *A. ceylanicum,* while two occur in cats, *A. tubaeforme* and *A. ceylanicum.* Two of these, *A. braziliense* and *A. ceylanicum* can develop in the small intestine of man but information on the differential frequencies and distribution in human, canine and feline hosts is confused owing to the taxonomic difficulties presented by this genus[40]. *A. ceylanicum* may be a natural parasite of man transmitted to his companion animals.

All these species are capable of invading the tissues of their natural hosts by skin penetration, although *Uncinaria* can only complete its life cycle if the larvae are swallowed. If infective third stage larvae of *A. braziliensis*, *A. tubaeforme* or *U. stenocephala* come into contact with the skin of other animals, including man, they start upon a futile migration by burrowing a tortuous tunnel and provoking an erythematous inflammatory reaction. This condition is known as cutaneous *larva migrans* or creeping eruption and can be of considerable nuisance value in some warmer areas such as Florida and the Mississippi Gulf coast. There are few reports from temperate regions even though *Uncinaria* can undoubtedly provoke cutaneous *larva migrans*. Presumably this is because there is less likelihood of bare human skin contacting contaminated soil or herbage. The Scandinavian literature contains one remarkable example of skin involvement in a bedwetting labourer who slept with a dog which ran away during the investigation[41].

Dirofilaria

Dirofilaria immitis is the causal agent of canine heartworm disease which is one of the most important, if not the most important, medical condition of dogs in the USA. Infections are encountered in most wet tropical and subtropical climates as well as in some localized areas of southern Europe. Heartworm disease presents a particular challenge to the veterinary profession as accurate diagnosis and successful therapy demand great expertise and the application of a wide range of modern techniques.

For reasons as yet unknown, *D. immitis* seems to be extending its geographical range. Fifteen years ago heartworm disease in the USA appeared to be widespread at serious disease-producing levels only within 50 to 70 miles of the Atlantic and Gulf coasts south of New Jersey, but a rapidly increasing number of severe clinical cases have since been recorded in the northern states of the USA and adjoining parts of Canada[42] (Figure 8.11). A similar trend has been observed in Australia where heartworm has spread southwards into Victoria[43].

The 20–30 cm long adult worms live entwined in the right ventricle of the canine heart producing microfilariae (Figure 8.12) which are often numbered in tens of thousands per ml of venous blood. These develop to infective larvae when taken up by one of the 60 or so species of anopheline and culicine mosquitoes that are potentially capable of transmitting this disease from dog to dog.

Prior to 1961 most cases of dirofilariasis diagnosed in man involved the subcutaneous tissues and were attributed to the related species *D. repens* (found in

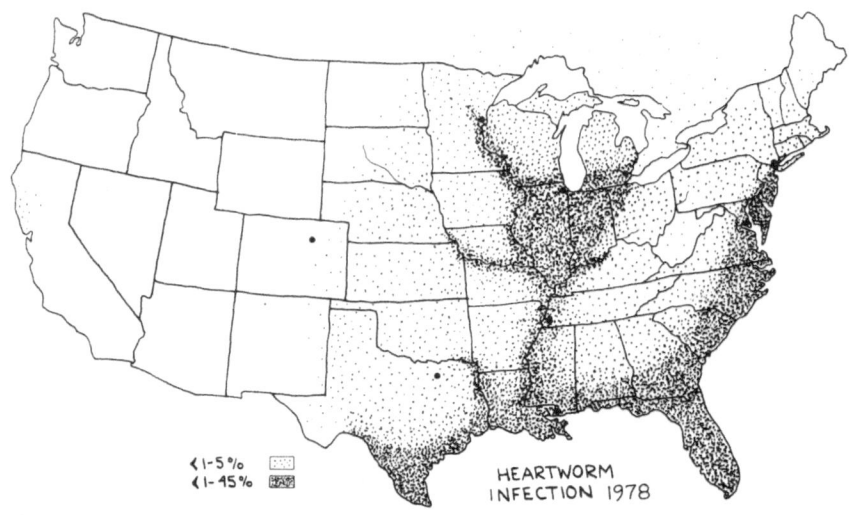

Figure 8.11 *Dirofilaria immitis*—extended zone of endemicity 1978 (Photograph American Heartworm Society)

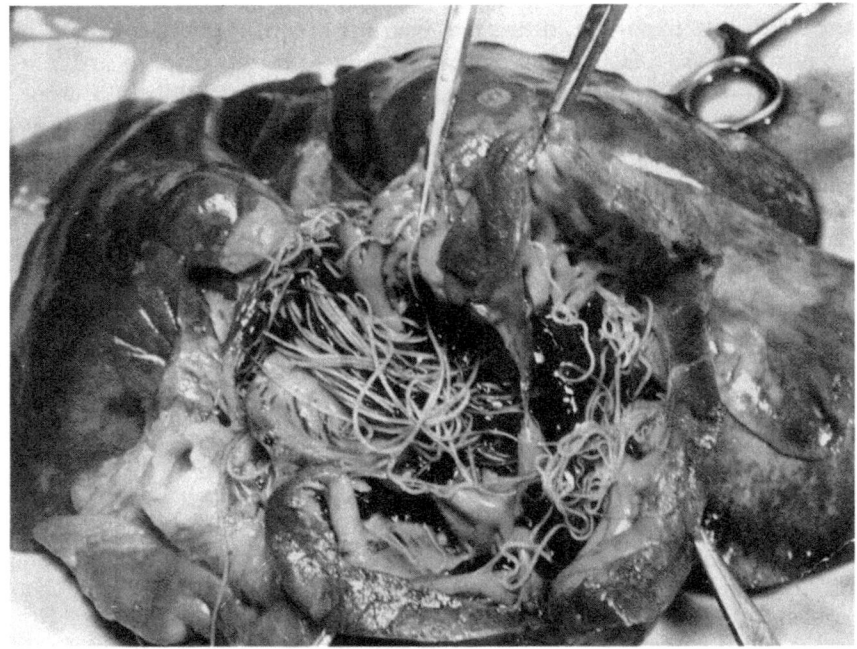

Figure 8.12 *Dirofilaria immitis* in heart of dog (Photograph American Heartworm Society)

dogs in the USSR and southern Europe[44]) or *D. tenuis* (normally parasitic in the racoon in the USA). After that date, the increasingly widespread use of mass radiography has led to the description of several dozen cases of pulmonary dirofilariasis, caused by *D. immitis*, in the USA, Australia, South America and Japan. Most infections are asymptomatic and discovered fortuitously, while the aetiology of some resected lesions may be overlooked as the worm is coiled or convoluted, occupying only a small part of the pathological mass.

The lesions are spherical, well delineated, non-calcified and solid, casting circular 'coin lesion' X-ray shadows with a diameter varying from several mm to several cm[45-47]. On histological examination, a degenerating immature worm can be seen within an arteriole surrounded by necrotic tissue enclosed in a fibrous reaction. It is as though *D. immitis* larvae from feeding mosquitoes migrate through the body of these individuals as they would in a dog but they fail to establish in the heart, being swept via the pulmonary artery to be entrapped in the lungs. Only one case has been reported of microfilariae being found in a human patient[48].

Trichuridae

This is a group of minor importance in the context of this chapter. Only one suspected instance of human infection with the dog whipworm, *Trichuris* (*Trichocephalus*) *vulpis*, is reported in the American literature but a prevalence of 6.1% has been claimed for kennel workers in Bucharest[49,50]. In view of the apparent ease with which the pig whipworm *T. suis* is established in man in experimental situations[51], it is possible that the canine species is on occasion overlooked as worms of this genus can only be differentiated by careful microscopic examination.

Nematodes of the genus *Capillaria* produce double-plugged eggs very similar to those of *Trichuris*. Two species with life cycles involving pet animals have been recovered from man on rare occasions. The first of these is *C. aerophila* which lives in the trachea and bronchi of foxes, mink and, less often, dogs and cats[52]. It has a simple direct life cycle. In contrast, the life history of *C. hepatica,* which lives in the liver of small mammals and very occasionally larger animals including man[53], is unique. The eggs accumulate in granulomatous lesions in the liver parenchyma. Transmission of infection can only occur after the death of the host animal. If it is eaten, the eggs are released from the hepatic tissues and pass through the intestine of the predator thereby gaining access to the environment. Thus, the role of the cat and dog, along with other carnivores, is to disseminate the infection although they themselves are rarely parasitized by this nematode.

Thelazia

Thelazia californiensis has a very restricted distribution, being found, as its name implies, in California and neighbouring states. The life cycle is uncertain but deer may be the main reservoir of infection and the deerfly the principal vector[54]. It is found in the conjunctival sac of dogs, cats, farm livestock and wild mammals, mainly in mountainous or unpopulated areas. Eight cases of conjunctivitis in humans attributable to this spiruroid nematode parasite had been reported up to 1975[55].

Gnathostoma

Another spiruroid, *Gnathostoma spinigerum*, is a relatively common cause of visceral and cutaneous *larva migrans* in some parts of south-east Asia, including Japan. It has also been reported in animals and man in Queensland[43]. Although this parasite is not related to *Spirometra*, the two life cycles have some similarities. Each uses the dog and cat as its final host, with *Cyclops* as the first intermediate host and a wide range of vertebrates as second intermediate hosts. Man is usually infected by eating raw or undercooked flesh containing encysted larvae.

Linguatula

The pentastomids, of which *Linguatula serrata* is a member, form a curious zoological group, worm-like in appearance but with some affinity to the arthropods. *L. serrata* is encountered infrequently in dogs and rarely in man. It inhabits the nasal cavities where it can grow to over 10 cm in length. It is tongue-shaped and its eggs, after being sneezed out of the body with nasal discharge, are taken up by herbivorous intermediate hosts. Nymphs encyst in the mesenteric lymph nodes and other organs awaiting ingestion by the definitive host.

Proud owners of pet pythons may be exposed to risk of abdominal pains caused by the pentastomid *Armillifer armillatus* transmitted in the snake's saliva or excreta[56].

Gasterophilus

The stomach bot is a dipteran that lays its eggs on the forelegs, lips or face of the horse. When licked into the mouth larvae from the eggs burrow into the buccal mucosa and make their way down the oesophagus to the stomach. Here they develop and when ready to pupate pass out of the host with the faeces.

If the eggs are deposited on human skin, the larvae may produce a form of cutaneous *larva migrans*.

A MISCELLANY

The final section of this chapter deals briefly with a number of parasitic conditions (most of which are fully described elsewhere in this book) in which the pet animal may be the victim as well as (or in some cases, rather than) the culprit.

Non-human primates share, or may be infected with, a number of human parasites including *Entamoeba, Giardia, Balantidium, Trichuris, Enterobius, Ancylostoma, Ascaris* and *Strongyloides*. Infection may be passed from ape to man or *vice versa*. Similarly, dogs may become infected with *Strongyloides stercoralis* and may on occasion act as a reservoir for human infection[57], but strongyloidiasis occurs only sporadically in the dog and most cases are attributed to canine rather than human strains of the parasite. The three protozoan species in the primate list have also been reported from dogs on rare occasions but it is doubtful if pet animals play any significant role in the epidemiology of these conditions.

Sometimes the zoonotic relationship between man and animals is reversed (when it is designated an anthroponosis) with man acting as the reservoir of infection that places the pets in his care at risk, as in the case of *Necator*, a human parasite which can 'accidentally' infect the dog. *Diphyllobothrium latum* might also be placed in this category as man is the main disseminator of this parasite. Dogs frequently harbour *D. latum* in endemic areas, but the tapeworm does not thrive in this host.

Lastly, both man and his companion animals may fall victim to parasites of other domestic or wild animals without there being more than a remote possibility of the pet transmitting the infection to his master or *vice versa*. Thus, both the horse and his rider can be infected with *Fasciola hepatica* while cats and dogs can harbour *Trichinella spiralis*. Some trematodes of foxes, mink and other wild mammals such as *Opisthorchis tenuicollis* and *Paragonimus kellicotti*, have been reported from dogs, cats and man, as has the acanthocephalan parasite of rodents, *Moniliformis moniliformis*.

Thus, there are many ways in which the world of parasites can interact with the life of man and his companion animals. Often the threads of this interplay weave patterns of extraordinary complexity. The examples given in this chapter are those that are most likely to be encountered in the Western World. The list is by no means comprehensive or definitive as new associations have been discovered in recent years and it is possible that there are others of which we are not yet aware. For example, a newly-discovered mange mite, *Trixacarus (Caviacoptes) caviae* is now known to be the cause of an intensely pruritic condition in pet guinea pigs[58]. It might be anticipated that this ectoparasite would provoke skin lesions in man similar to those produced by *Sarcoptes scabiei* var. *canis*, although there is as yet no evidence to support this view. Man's increasing mobility and his desire to be accompanied by his pets can result in the importation of tropical and subtropical diseases such as leishmaniasis into temperate regions and the introduction of organisms such as *Dirofilaria* and *Rhipicephalus* into non-endemic areas. These dangers are, however, minimized in those countries with strict quarantine regulations. Man's propensity for keeping unusual pets will also cause the list of zoonotic parasitoses to swell, perhaps in an unpredictable and unexpected manner.

References

1. Levinson, B. M. (1975). Pets and environment. In: Anderson, R. S. (ed.). *Pet Animals and Society*. pp. 8–18 (London: Balliere Tindall)
2. Carding, A. (1975). The growth of pet population in Western Europe and the implications for dog control in Great Britain. In: Anderson, R. S. (ed.). *Pet Animals and Society*. pp. 66–88 (London: Balliere Tindall)
3. Jenner, E. (1798). *An enquiry into the cause and effects of the variolae vaccinae*. p. 2. (London: Published by the author)
4. Walters, T. M. H. (1978). Hydatid disease in Wales: 1. Epidemiology. *Vet. Record*, **102**, 257
5. Clarkson, M. J. (1978). Hydatid disease in Wales: 2. Eradication. *Vet. Record*, **102**, 259
6. Thompson, R. C. A. (1977). Hydatidosis in Great Britain. *Helminthol. Abstr.*, **46**, 837
7. Lukashenko, N. P. (1971). Problems of epidemiology and prophylaxis of alveococcosis (multilocular echinococcosis): a general review—with particular reference to the USSR. *Int. J. Parasitol.*, **1**, 125
8. Bisseru, B., Woodruff, A. W. and Hutchinson, R. W. (1966). Infection with adult *Toxocara canis*. *Br. Med. J.*, **1**, 1583
9. Nichols, R. L. (1956). The aetiology of *visceral larva migrans*. 1. Diagnostic morphology of infective second-stage *Toxocara* larvae. *J. Parasitol.*, **42**, 349
10. Stevenson, P. (1978). *A study of larval ascarid infections of pigs and their importance as a cause of liver pathology in Great Britain*. Ph.D. Thesis. University of London
11. Beaver, P. C. (1969). The nature of *visceral larva migrans*. *J. Parasitol.*, **55**, 3
12. Schantz, P. M. and Glickman, L. T. (1978). Current concepts in Parasitology: Toxocaral *visceral larva migrans*. *N. Engl. J. Med.*, **298**, 436
13. Woodruff, A. W. (1970). Toxocariasis. *Br. Med. J.*, **3**, 663
14. Woodruff, A. W. (1978). Restriction on dogs (correspondence). *The London Times*, 12th January, 1978
15. Jacobs, D. E., Pegg, E. J. and Stevenson, P. (1977). Helminths of British dogs: *Toxocara canis*—a veterinary perspective. *J. Small Animal Practice*, **18**, 79
16. Ghadirian, E., Viens, P., Strykowski, H. and Dubreuil, F. (1976). Epidemiology of toxocariasis in the Montreal area. Prevalence of *Toxocara* and other helminths in dogs and soil. *Can. J. Publ. Hlth.*, **67**, 495
17. Jacobs, D. E., Woodruff, A. W., Shah, A. I. and Prole, J. H. B. (1977). *Toxocara* infections and kennel workers. *Br. Med. J.*, **1**, 51
18. Frenkel, J. K. (1973). Toxoplasmosis: Parasite life cycle, pathology and immunology. In: Hammond, D. M. and Long, P. L. (eds). *The Coccidia: Eimeria, Isospora, Toxoplasma and Related Genera*, pp. 343–410. (Baltimore: University Park Press and London: Butterworths)
19. Dubey, J. P. (1977). *Toxoplasma, Hammondia, Besnoitia, Sarcocystis* and other cyst-forming coccidia of man and animals. In: Kreier, J. P. (ed.). *Parasitic Protozoa. Volume 3: Gregarines, Haemogregarines, Coccidia, Plasmodia and Haemoproteids*, pp. 101–237. (New York: Academic Press)
20. Beverley, J. K. A. (1976). Toxoplasmosis in animals. *Vet. Record*, **99**, 123
21. Dubey, J. P. (1973). Feline toxoplasmosis and coccidiosis: a survey of domiciled and stray cats. *J. Am. Vet. Med. Assoc.*, **162**, 873
22. Wallace, G. D. (1973). The role of the cat in the natural history of *Toxoplasma gondii*. *Am. J. Trop. Med. Hyg.*, **22**, 313
23. Frenkel, J. K. (1975). Toxoplasmosis in cats and man. *Feline Practice*, **5**, 28
24. Hewitt, M., Walton, G. S. and Waterhouse, M. (1971). Pet animal infestations and human

skin lesions. *Br. J. Dermatol.,* **85,** 215
25. Beresford-Jones, W. P. (1978). Personal communication
26. Kissileff, A. (1938). The dog flea as a causative agent in summer eczema. *J. Am. Vet. Med. Assoc.,* **46,** 21
27. Baker, K. P. and Hatch, C. (1972). The species of fleas found on Dublin dogs. *Vet. Record,* **91,** 151
28. Mourier, H. (1976). Cat and dog fleas: life history and control. *Dansk Veterinaer-tidsskrift,* **59,** 581
29. Winding, O., Willeberg. P. and Haarlov, N. (1970). The brown dog tick (*Rh. sanguineus*), an ectoparasite of dogs of current interest. *Nordisk Veterinaermedicin,* **22,** 48
30. Gregor, W. W. (1965). The incidence of skin disease in small animal practice. In: Rook, A. J. and Walton, G. S. (eds). *Comparative Physiology and Pathology of the Skin,* pp. 33–70 (Oxford: Blackwell)
31. Thomsett, L. R. (1968). Mite infestations of man contracted from dogs and cats. *Br. Med. J.,* **3,** 93
32. Gething, M. A. (1973). *Cheyletiella* infestation in small animals. *Vet. Bull.,* **43,** 63
33. Williams, B. M. (1976). The epidemiology of adult and larval (tissue) cestodes in Dyfed (UK) 1. The cestodes of farm dogs. *Vet. Parasitol.* **1,** 271
34. Hermos, J. A., Healy, G. R., Schultz, M. G., Barlow, J. and Chard, W. G. (1970). Fatal human cerebral coenurosis. *J. Am. Med. Assoc.,* **213,** 1461
35. Templeton, A. C. (1971). Anatomical and geographical location of human coenurus infection. *Trop. Geogr. Med.,* **23,** 105
36. Sterba, J., Blazek, K. and Barus, V. (1977). Contribution to the pathology of strobilocercosis (*Strobilocerus fasciolaris*) in the liver of man and some animals. *Folia Parasitol.,* **24,** 41
37. Schwartzwelder, J. C., Beaver, P. C. and Hood, M. W. (1964). Sparganosis in southern United States. *Am. J. Trop. Med. Hyg.,* **13,** 43
38. Moore, D. V. and Connell, F. H. (1960) Additional records of *Dipylidium caninum* infections in children in the United States with observations on treatment. *Am. J. Trop. Med. Hyg.,* **9,** 604
39. Kelley, J. D. (1977). *Canine Parasitology. Veterinary Review No. 17.* (Sydney: University of Sydney Postgraduate Foundation in Veterinary Science)
40. Miller, T. A. (1971). Vaccination against the canine hookworm diseases. In: Dawes, B. (ed.). *Advances in Parasitology, Volume 9,* pp. 153–183 (London & New York: Academic Press)
41. Astrup, A. (1945). *Uncinaria stenocephala* as a cause of disease in man. *Acta Dermato-venereol.,* **25,** 389
42. Otto, G. F. (1975). Changing geographic distribution of heartworm disease in the United States. In: Morgan, H. C. (ed.). *Proceedings of the Heartworm Symposium, 1974,* pp. 1–2 (Bonner Springs, Kansas: VM Publishing Inc.)
43. Kelley, J. D. (1974). Anthropozoönotic helminthiases in Australia. The role of animals in disease transmission. *Int. J. Zoonoses,* **1,** 1
44. Carneri, I. de, Sacchi, S. and Pazzaglia, A. (1973). Subcutaneous dirofilariasis in man—not so rare. *Trans. Roy. Soc. Trop. Med. Hyg.,* **67,** 887
45. Neafie, R. C. and Piggott, M. A. J. J. (1971). Human pulmonary dirofilariasis. *Arch. Pathol.,* **92,** 342
46. Pierson, K. K. (1972). Gumma-like pulmonary granulomas due to *Dirofilaria* sp. in man. In: Bradley, R. E. and Pacheco, F. H. (eds.) *Canine Heartworm Disease,* pp. 33–37 (Gainsville, Fla.: University of Florida Press)
47. Moorhouse, D. E., Abrahams, E. W. and Stephens, B. J. (1971). Human pulmonary dirofilariasis in Queensland. *Med. J. Austr.,* **2,** 1230
48. Greene, B. M. (1975). Microfilaraemia in a patient with systemic lupus erythematosus: case report. In: Morgan, H. C. (ed.). *Proceedings of the Heartworm Symposium 1974,* pp. 14–15 (Bonner Springs, Kansas: VM Publishing inc.)
49. Hall, J. E. and Sonnenberg, B. (1956). An apparent case of human infection with the whipworm of dogs, *Trichuris vulpis* (Froelich, 1789). *J. Parasitol.,* **42,** 197
50. Dinulescu, G., Stoenescu, D., Ricman, T. *et al.* (1975). Observations on the frequency of various helminthiases in man and their connexion with helminthiases in dogs. *Trop. Dis. Bull. Lon.,* (1958), **55,** 902 (Abstract)

51. Beer, R. J. S. (1976). The relationship between *Trichuris trichiura* (Linnaeus 1758) of man and *Trichuris suis* (Schrank 1788) of the pig. *Res. Vet. Sci.*, **20**, 47

52. Coudert, J., Despeignes, J. and Battesti, M. R. (1972). A propos d'un cas de capillariose pulmonaire. *Bull. Soci. Pathol. Exot.*, **65**, 841

53. Otto. G. F., Berthrong, M., Appleby, R. E. and Wilbur, O. (1954). Eosinophilia and hepatomegaly due to *Capillaria hepatica* infection. *Bull. Johns Hopkins Hosp.*, **94**, 319

54. Schauffler, A. F. (1966). Canine thelaziasis in Arizona. *J. Am. Vet. Med. Assoc.*, **149**, 521

55. Knierim, R. and Jack, M. K. (1975). Conjunctivitis due to *Thelazia californiensis*. *Arch. Ophthalmol.*, **93**, 522

56. Cohen, D. (1975). Zoonoses in perspective. In: Anderson, R. S. (ed.). *Pet Animals and Society*, pp. 139–154 (London: Balliere Tindall)

57. Georgi, J. R. and Sprinkle, C. L. (1974). A case of human strongyloidosis apparently contracted from asymptomatic colony dogs. *Am. J. Trop. Med. Hyg.*, **23**, 899

58. Thoday, K. L. and Beresford-Jones, W. P. (1977). The diagnosis and treatment of mange in the guinea-pig caused by *Trixacarus (Caviacoptes) caviae* (Fain, Hovell and Hyatt, 1972). *J. Small Animal Practice*, **18**, 591

General texts

Hoeden, J. van der. (1964). *Zoonoses*. (Amsterdam: Elsevier)

Bisseru, B. (1967). *Diseases of Man acquired from his Pets*. (London: Balliere Tindall)

Hubbert, W. T., McCulloch, W. F. and Schnurrenburger, P. R. (1975). *Diseases transmitted from Animals to Man*. (Springfield, Illinois: Charles C. Thomas)

9
Man and Domestic Animals

T. E. GIBSON

INTRODUCTION

Domestic farm animals such as cattle, horses, sheep, pigs and poultry may carry a great variety of protozoan, helminth or arthropod parasites. Although many of these cause considerable financial losses to farmers, fortunately relatively few constitute a hazard to man. The dangers from direct contact with animals are very slight and are mainly from arthropod parasites which may transfer temporarily to man. The risk here is mainly an occupational one (to farm workers), although ticks and red mites of poultry may be acquired from the environment without direct contact with animals. The majority of the protozoan parasites of farm animals are not transmitted to man but *Babesia* species are the exception, being transmitted by the bites of ticks which have become infected by feeding on infected cattle. None of the helminth parasites are transmitted from animals to man by direct contact. The most important danger to man from this group is from parasites which either use both man and domestic animals as alternative hosts or those in which man in addition to one of the domestic animals serves as host for different parts of the life cycle. In these two categories three important parasites are found: *Trichinella spiralis*, *Taenia saginata* and *Taenia solium*. Other parasites which are often found in domestic animals and occasionally infect man include *Hypodema* species and *Fasciola hepatica*.

In this chapter, the parasites of importance to Western man, by virtue of his habit of rearing domestic animals to provide him with food and clothing, are dealt with under three main headings: arthropod parasites, protozoan parasites and helminthic parasites.

ARTHROPOD PARASITES

Arthropod parasites are generally host-specific but a few of those found on domestic animals are able to transfer to man and survive for varying periods of

201

time. The mite *Sarcoptes scabiei* transfers readily from the dog and the fox to
the horse. Man may become infested from any of these three sources and the
parasites burrow into the skin to produce lesions typical of human scabies. The
sheep ked, *Melophagus ovinus*, readily transfers from sheep to man and
remains on the skin or in clothing for several days. It causes no discomfort and
there is no evidence that it will bite the human host. Lice of various species are
found on cattle, goats, sheep and poultry and although they will infest man, do
not bite the skin and hence live only for a few days. Fleas from poultry also infest man and it is generally accepted that they will bite, but they rarely become
established.

Human beings may also become infested with ticks. The life cycle of the tick
is acted out on the ground in the herbage mat. An illustrative life cycle is that of
Ixodes ricinus (sheep tick), the eggs of which are laid in crevices in the ground
and other sheltered places. The rate of development depends on the
temperature and usually development of the larva is not complete until the end
of August in temperate climates. From then until October larvae hatch out
from the eggs. These larvae usually remain inactive during the winter months
but in the spring of the following year they climb to the tips of grasses and
other plants where they wait for a suitable host to pass through. When opportunity affords the larva latches on to a suitable host, feeds for three to six days,
and then drops off to return to the herbage. During this, their second summer
of life, they moult and become nymphs. These remain inactive during the
autumn and winter and again in the spring climb the herbage, attach to a
suitable host and feed as the larvae did the previous year. After three to five
days feeding they drop off into the herbage and during the summer of the third
year moult to become adults. The adults follow the same pattern of quiescence
during the winter and in spring locate a host, feed and return to the herbage so
that the cycle can begin again. The larva, nymph and adult are all capable of at-
taching to a human being in mistake for their animal host (usually cattle).

The attached arthropod sucks blood and produces an inflamed lesion which
causes considerable irritation. The ticks are capable of passing on to man
parasites they normally transmit to cattle and a number of recorded cases of
Babesia infection have arisen in this way.

Red mites, *Dermanyssus gallinae*, of poultry will desert poultry houses from
which the birds have been removed and may be seen moving about on the outside. They can migrate to human beings and cause infestations but there is little
evidence that they bite man. Red mites are very uncommon in poultry houses
under modern conditions. Wild birds however are commonly infested with red
mites, as are their nests. Dwellings can be invaded by swarms of mites which
have left nests which are attached to the house and have been deserted by
birds. In this way infestation arises in man. The northern fowl mite, *Liponyssus
sylviarum* can also be found in large numbers on poultry and may infect man
but does not pierce the skin and seldom lives longer than a few days.

Another arthropod parasite which occasionally attacks man is the cattle warble fly, of which two species, *Hypoderma bovis* and *H. lineatum,* occur in Britain. The warble fly usually lays its eggs on the skin of the legs and lower abdomen of cattle. The larvae which hatch from the egg penetrate the skin and undertake a complex migration through the tissues of the host to finally reach the back. Here they produce a characteristic swelling known as the 'warble'. This swelling is open and from it the larvae leave the host to pupate on the ground. Occasionally, warble flies lay eggs on human beings in which case the larvae penetrate the skin. There is some evidence that they migrate through human tissues since infected individuals often describe irritation, pain and discomfort in various sites before the warble appears on the skin. The definitive evidence that a patient is infected with larvae of the warble fly is a reddenned, raised, slightly tender area on the skin which ultimately bursts releasing a small white maggot which can be identified by an entomologist as *Hypoderma* species. A patient can be infected with several larvae at one time, there is no specific treatment and the condition is self-limiting with resolution of the skin lesion following liberation of the larva.

PROTOZOAN PARASITES

Protozoan diseases are generally host-specific although infections with *Babesia* species derived from animals have been reported on a few occasions in man. The *Babesia* are blood parasites and are transmitted from one mammalian host to another by the bite of a tick. Accidental infection in man can arise from the bite of a tick infected with *Babesia*. Three cases of human babesiosis, presumably derived from cattle, have been reported from Yugoslavia, California and Eire. In the third case the organism involved was specifically identified as *Babesia divergens*. These cases all occurred in splenectomized individuals and two of them were fatal. An investigation carried out in Eire failed to detect *Babesia* antibodies in 36 persons who had intact spleens. The disease was initially diagnosed as malaria, suggested by the symptoms of chills, fever, headache and lethargy. Examination of blood smears, however, revealed the presence of *Babesia* organisms not *Plasmodium*. No satisfactory treatment is known but it has been suggested that the veterinary preparation amicarbalide (Diampron) could be used at a dose of 10 mg per kg.

Although not strictly relevant to the consideration of infections derived from domestic animals it is of interest to note that six cases of babesiosis have been diagnosed on Nantucket Island in persons having intact spleens. The symptoms were similar to those described above. Examination of blood smears revealed that the *Babesia* involved were of rodent origin.

HELMINTHIC PARASITES

Trichinella spiralis

This nematode infects man and a wide range of carnivorous mammals. The pig, rat and various wild carnivores are the most frequently infected, although many other species have been experimentally infected. Experimental infections have also been produced in birds. In most western countries the pig is the most important source of infection for man but wild boars, bears and other game animals are frequent sources of infection in countries where hunting is popular.

Geographical distribution

Human infections occur sporadically in Canada as a result of eating uncooked sausage and similar food. Recent surveys in which diaphragms from randomly selected cadavers were examined showed *T. spiralis* to be present in 4–6% in British Columbia, 2% in Toronto, and 1.5% in Montreal. Numerous surveys of the prevalence of the condition in pigs have revealed infection rates of 4–5% in Vancouver, 6.5% in Toronto, 2% in Montreal and 0.4% in the Maritime Provinces. In Arctic Canada the prevalence is very high. In some areas 95% of the population are affected.

In the USA a marked decrease in the prevalence in man has been noted in recent years, associated with the introduction of the compulsory boiling of swill before it is fed to pigs. Surveys carried out between 1931 and 1950 revealed a prevalence varying from 2.9% to 36%, whereas between 1957 and 1958 a much lower level was recorded (1–5.0% with an average of 4.1%). The prevalence in swill-fed animals has shown a dramatic decline. In 1950 a survey showed 11% of pigs fed raw swill to be infected but after the introduction of cooked swill this figure was reduced to 2.2% between 1954–1959. A more recent survey carried out between 1964 and 1966 showed the prevalence to have decreased even further to 0.5%.

In Europe the diagnosis of trichinosis in pigs has been made by the trichinoscope which is a less sensitive method than the digestion technique. The data on prevalence in Europe cannot therefore be compared with that from North America. It is, however, evident that the prevalence in most European countries is low. Many countries, including Switzerland, Belgium, Holland, Denmark and the UK, claim that their pig population is virtually free from *T. spiralis*. Countries which appear to have higher rates of infection are Rumania and Greece, but from a number of countries such as Albania data are almost non-existent. There are reports of human infection from most European countries and it is noteworthy that a high prevalence can occur in the human population in countries where prevalence amongst pigs is low. Germany, for example, during the second half of the 19th century suffered severe epidemics, when only 0.05% of slaughtered pigs were found to be infected. Following the introduction of trichinoscopy, the prevalence fell rapidly to 0.001% in 1926 and by 1966 was 0.000028%. Today it is uncommon to discover an infected pig in the abattoir. The occurrence of severe outbreaks of trichinosis in man, in the face of a low prevalence amongst pigs could be explained by the popularity in the German diet of foods containing raw or partially cooked pork. In England outbreaks in the human population have occurred sporadically, the last in the civilian population occurring in 1967. The most recent survey of infection (carried out by digesting pieces of diaphragm) revealed a prevalence of 0.4% and the general impression is that this low prevalence is an accurate reflection of the problem. In the 1940s surveys of prevalence in pigs in Great Britain failed to reveal any animals carrying infection. It must be concluded that in Britain trichinosis in pigs does not occur or at least is extremely rare and that infection in man is very unusual.

In Russia *T. spiralis* infection in pigs is not uniformly distributed, the areas where the highest levels of infection occur being Byelorussia, the Ukraine and the foothills of the Caucasus. About one million pigs from central Russia are slaughtered annually in Moscow and the prevalence of trichinosis has been found to be 8–30 per 10 000. Outbreaks in man have been sporadic and related to the consumption of uninspected pork or infected wild animals. The highest infection rate is seen in Byelorussia, where surveys have revealed 1.36% of the population to be infected. No severe epidemics have been recorded in Russia, although in isolated communities outbreaks involving up to 50 people have occurred, with some fatalities.

Although a number of individuals in Australia have been found to be infected with *T. spiralis*, all of them were born outside the continent. There is no firm evidence to suggest that the infection is endemic in Australia. In New Zealand *T. spiralis* is present but at a very low level.

Control

Control is most effectively achieved by limiting the opportunities for pigs to acquire infection. The main source of infection for pigs is swill and in the United States the obligatory boiling of swill resulted in a marked decrease in the prevalence of trichinosis in pigs as has been previously discussed. Pigs may acquire infection from rats, foxes or other wildlife, but these sources are of minor importance under modern rearing conditions. Nevertheless, the elimination of vermin from pig houses is a sensible action to take for a variety of reasons.

A number of countries rely on the trichinoscope as a screening tool to prevent the release on the market of infected pork. After slaughter a sample of pig diaphragm is removed, cut into sixteen pieces (each about the size of an oatgrain) and placed on a special slide which enables them to be compressed and examined under the microscope. Special projection microscopes are available in abattoirs, where regular examination for *T. spiralis* is undertaken, but an ordinary low power microscope is a satisfactory alternative (Figure 9.1). Recent work has revealed that trichinoscope examination misses a proportion of lightly infected pigs. In an experiment to compare the efficiency of the trichinoscope with the techniques of artificial digestion of meat and the fluorescent antibody test, it was found that light infections initiated by administering 50 larvae to the animal were not detected by any of the methods. Heavier infections,

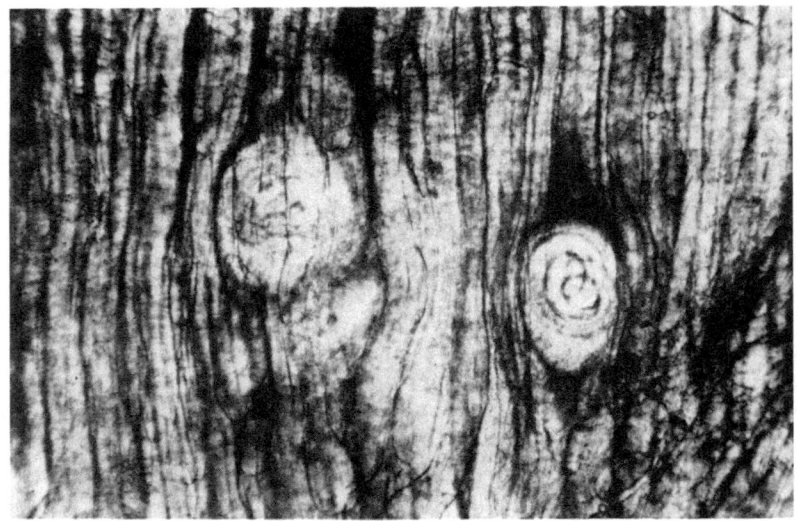

Figure 9.1   *Trichinella spiralis* in muscle

produced by 150 larvae, could be detected by both digestion and fluorescent antibody tests but the trichinoscope only detected infections produced by 500 larvae or more. Thus trichinoscope examination results give a false sense of security to the consumer, (especially in countries where uncooked pork is used in meat products) because meat certified as free from *Trichinella* may still be lightly infected.

Digestion using pepsin is a more efficient method of screening samples of meat for the presence of *Trichinella* and is in routine use, for example, in Denmark. One-gram samples are grouped together in hundreds for digestion, and placed in a 1% pepsin 0.5% HCl solution and incubated at 37 °C for 4–6 hours. The *Trichinella* larvae are recovered from the digest by screening and sedimentation. This long process is inconvenient for routine abattoir use and the Danes have devised a new digestion technique using an apparatus called a 'stomacher' which accelerates the process so that the examination may be completed in one hour. If larvae are found in one of the bulk samples then it is necessary to examine each individual sample from that batch of a hundred to identify the infected animal. The technique is most practicable in countries where *Trichinella* is absent or rarely found, to monitor the continued low prevalence of the infection.

Serological tests, such as the fluorescent antibody test or the more efficient ELISA test, although not suitable for use in the abattoir, are useful tools in survey work. The latter test is especially appropriate for surveys of prevalence as it can be carried out with automated equipment.

Pork which is found to be infected with *Trichinella* may be rendered safe for human consumption by refrigeration. Various refrigeration regimens have been suggested and it has been found that the temperature is not important providing the time of refrigeration is appropriate. A suitable regimen is as follows: prior to having been placed in the freezer the meat should have been chilled to between 0 and 2 °C. The chilled meat is then placed in a freezing room at −25 °C, the duration of its stay in the freezer depending on its thickness. Meat under 25 cm in thickness should remain at −25 °C for at least 240 hours, pieces 25–50 cm thick should remain 480 hours. Pieces thicker than 50 cm must first be cut into smaller sections before freezing.

Smoking, salting and drying used in the production of sausage and other pork products will in many cases destroy *T. spiralis* larvae although not all curing processes are adequate and some countries maintain lists of approved curing processes. It is unwise to rely on curing processes alone to destroy *T. spiralis* and pork used in the preparation of sausages and other products should be known to be free from *Trichinella* or should be treated by refrigeration or cooking prior to use. The larvae of *T. spiralis* are rapidly killed at 55 °C and the US Bureau of Animal Industry requires that pork or pork products which are to be consumed without further cooking should be heated to 58.3 °C during processing.

In the home, adequate cooking of pork and pork products is an important safeguard against human infection. It is important that the centre of the meat should reach an adequate temperature and this is not necessarily ensured by keeping the oven at that temperature. (A temperature of 60 °C should be achieved in cooking pork.) A large joint may therefore require several hours' cooking in order to reach that critical temperature in its middle. The colour of the juice exuding from the meat is a useful indicator. If it is grey or brown the meat will have reached a temperature of 80 °C and will be safe. The frying of bacon or ham will also destroy the parasites.

Taenia saginata

It has been estimated that some 39 millions of the world's population are infected with *Taenia saginata* but these are mainly in Africa. The adult tapeworm lives in the small intestine of man and gravid segments are passed in the faeces. Each segment may contain 100 000 eggs. When eggs are swallowed by a bovine animal they hatch, liberating an oncosphere which migrates into the gut wall and so gains entrance to the blood and lymph vessels. Eggs are carried by the circulatory system to the striated muscles especially those of the tongue, neck, shoulder and hind limbs and also heart muscles. In the muscle the egg develops to a cysticerus (*Cysticercus bovis*) reaching its full size in about 12 to 15 weeks (Figure 9.2). Mature cysts when ingested by man in uncooked meat develop into a tapeworm in the intestine. Cysts begin to degenerate shortly after maturity is reached and it is often possible to find both

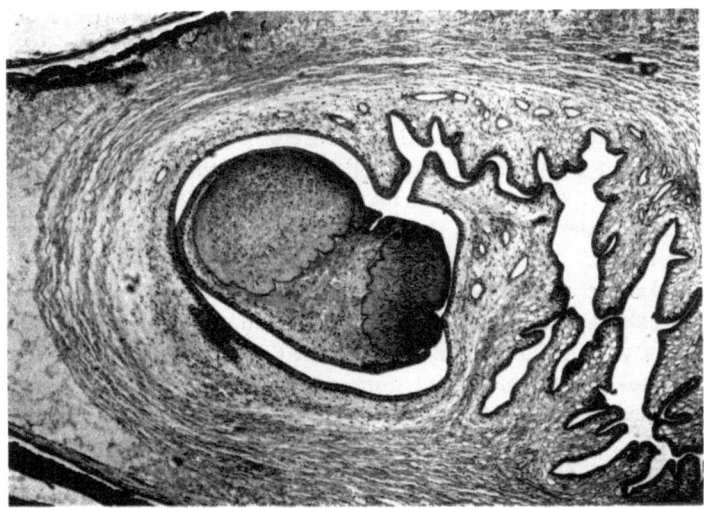

Figure 9.2 Section of viable *C. bovis*. Within the thin outer cuticle is seen a layer of contractile fibres, some transverse and some longitudinal, forming a network. Within this network is the nucleate parenchymatous tissue, in which muscle- and nerve-cells can be recognized. Numerous calcareous corpuscles can be seen in the parenchymatous tissue, particularly in the neck region. (Haematoxylin and eosin.) (×37 approx.)

viable and degenerate cysts within the same animal. Man is infested solely by consuming infected meat in the raw state. There is no occupational hazard to farm workers.

Geographical distribution

A survey of the prevalence of *Cysticercus bovis* in slaughtered cattle shows it to be uncommon in most countries in Europe. Prevalence is under 1% except in Czechoslovakia (4.5%), Germany (4%), Greece (3%) and Switzerland (4.9%). Similarly in Canada, USA, Australia and New Zealand, the parasite is rare or absent. Countries with a high prevalence (over 10%) include Congo Republic, Eritrea, Guinea, Kenya, Libya, Nigeria, Dubangi, Sierra Leone, Swaziland, Uganda, Mexico, Azerbaijan, Bali, Syria and parts of Russia and Yugoslavia. Other countries in which *C. bovis* is reported to be common are Angola, Somalia, the Ivory Coast, Tanganyika, Argentina, Chile, Costa Rica, Peru, Afghanistan, Burma, Laos and Albania. The majority of these countries are those where hygiene is poor and opportunities for the infection of cattle from human excreta are thus numerous.

Control

Four aspects of control measures need to be considered:

(a) Control of infections in man.

(b) Hygiene and efficient sewage disposal.

(c) Efficient meat inspection to reduce the chances of transmission to man.

(d) The treatment of infected meat to render it safe for human consumption.

(a) Control of infection in man

Each gravid segment of *T. saginata* contains about 100 000 eggs so that human excreta is a potent source of infection to cattle. The tapeworm causes few ill effects in man and formerly when treatment was unpleasant many carriers were reluctant to comply with the regime. In some primitive societies the presence of a tapeworm is regarded as a sign of manhood and treatment is not welcomed. Nowadays efficient cestodicides, free of side effects, are available and there is no longer any reason why human beings should be tapeworm carriers.

(b) Control by sewage disposal

In primitive societies sanitary arrangements may be non-existent and human faeces regularly contaminate the grazing grounds of cattle. In such circumstances a considerable meaure of control can be achieved by the installation of latrines, the use of which minimizes or even eliminates the contamination of cattle grazing areas and so reduces the general level of infection.

The sewage systems of advanced countries are very effective in reducing the contamination of the environment with infected faeces, but there is ample evidence that many sewage systems allow helminth eggs to pass into the effluent. In many seaside towns sewage is discharged into the sea without treatment and, moreover, the situation of the outfalls and the effect of currents may result in the deposition of faecal matter on beaches. It has been observed that seagulls ingest faeces deposited in this way and since tapeworm eggs may pass through their gastrointestinal tract unharmed, seagulls may therefore carry infection to inland pastures.

Tapeworm eggs are quite capable of passing through the filtration systems of ordinary sewage works and may therefore pass out with the effluent. Cattle can become infected by the ingestion of eggs along with the herbage of pastures contaminated with effluent. Some eggs find their way into the sewage sludge and will not be killed in air dried sludge unless it has been stored for one year. Sludge which has undergone mesophilic digestion or cold digestion in lagoons for 18 months is safe to use on grassland. In some modern sewage works mechanical filtration using 'microstraining' devices are employed. A very pure effluent results from this process and 90% of *Taenia* ova are retained. Most rural sewage disposal systems are of the type that the contamination of pastures is likely either due to overflowing of septic tanks or to the discharge of effluent into streams bordering on grazing land. If all sewage systems could be raised to the standard of the most efficient the possibility of contamination of pasture with *Taenia* eggs by effluent or sludge would be minimal. The capital cost of such an undertaking is not justified simply to control *Taenia saginata* but improvements in sewage works as they are replaced or extended will serve this purpose.

(c)   The role of meat inspection

Cysts may be found in any part of a bovine carcass and it would not be possible to be sure that *C. bovis* were absent unless every muscle had been subjected to multiple incision. This is clearly incompatible with the level of production of prime quality beef and some compromise must be arrived at which will reveal the majority of infected carcasses without seriously mutilating those not infected. Experience has shown that the majority of infected carcasses will be detected if incisions are made into the external masseter muscles from the lower border of the jaw, with a single incision into the internal masseter muscle. An additional incision is made into the left ventricle exposing its inner surface which may also be incised if necessary. Many meat inspectors also routinely incise the pillars of the diaphragm and palpate the tongue. Some authorities have also advocated cuts into the shoulder and hind limb but these increase the spoilage rate and the routine adoption of these added measures is not justified.

The cyst when exposed in incised muscle is easily recognizable. It is 6–9 mm in length and about 5 mm in diameter, and the scolex is readily seen as a white spot within the cyst. Further confirmation of the identity of the cyst is obtained by examination of the crushed cyst under the low power of the microscope when the scolex bearing four suckers will be seen. Degenerated cysts present more difficulty, but are generally similar in size and shape but contain a yellow caseous mass. A cyst which has calcified usually shrinks in size so that there is no positive means of identification.

Some continental authorities advocate the use of ultraviolet light to assist the detection of cysts in the meat. The cysts are visible as red fluorescent bodies on a blue–black background. There is little evidence, however, that this method improves the detection rate sufficiently to warrant the extra effort and expense involved in its use.

The action to be taken when *C. bovis* is detected in meat is laid down in the meat inspection regulations of various countries. Usually regulations require that cases of generalized infection are condemned as unfit for human consumption. When infection is localized the affected part only is condemned and the rest placed in cold storage (at −7 °C for three weeks or −10 °C for two weeks).

(d)   Control by other means

The use of refrigeration to render meat safe for human consumption has already been discussed. The exact temperature is not critical providing the time of exposure of the meat to that temperature is sufficient. Cooking destroys the cysticerci and temperatures similar to those recommended for *T. spiralis* are suitable. The habit of eating beef steak partially cooked or consuming certain dishes containing raw beef is fraught with danger.

Taenia solium

It has been estimated that some 2.5 millions of the world's population carry *Taenia solium*, the majority of these being in Africa. The adult parasites, 2–17 metres in length, inhabit the small intestine of man. Gravid segments passed in human faeces contain eggs which are immediately infective. When ingested by a pig, a migration similar to that described for *Taenia saginata* takes place and the cysts which develop in the muscles of pigs infect man when he consumes undercooked pork. If the eggs are consumed by man, similar migration to that occurring in the pig takes place and cysts will develop in the musculature and other sites including the brain.

Geographical distribution

In Europe, USA, Canada, Australia and New Zealand, *T. solium* is rare or even absent. It is however common in central Europe, India, China, Africa and Mexico.

Control

Control is essentially similar to that described for *Taenia saginata*. The control of human cysticercosis essentially concerns personal hygiene. Infected persons should be treated with an appropriate anthelminthic to prevent autoinfection by retroperistalsis and contaminated fingers. If sanitary facilities are poor, vegetables should always be washed and cooked before being eaten.

Fasciola hepatica (liver fluke)

This is a parasite of great importance in sheep, cattle, pigs and to a lesser extent in horses but it can develop successfully in many other mammals including man. The life cycle of the liver fluke is complex. The adult fluke (Figure 9.3) lives in the bile ducts of cattle, sheep and other hosts and the eggs laid by the fluke pass down the bile ducts into the intestine and reach the exterior in the faeces. Development takes place within the egg and a free living larva called a miracidium develops. This larva is capable of swimming in the thin film of water which covers the soil in damp places and in this way it reaches and penetrates a snail of the species *Limnaea truncatula* in which further development takes place. Several larval stages are undertaken in the snail and when the final stage (cercaria) is reached it leaves the snail and swims on to blades of grass and other vegetation where it encysts. These cysts are swallowed in the herbage by grazing sheep or cattle and pass down the intestine of these animals where the cyst wall is digested. This process liberates a young fluke which penetrates the wall of the intestine and migrates across the abdominal cavity to reach the liver. It penetrates the liver and burrows through the parenchyma to reach a bile duct, where it matures.

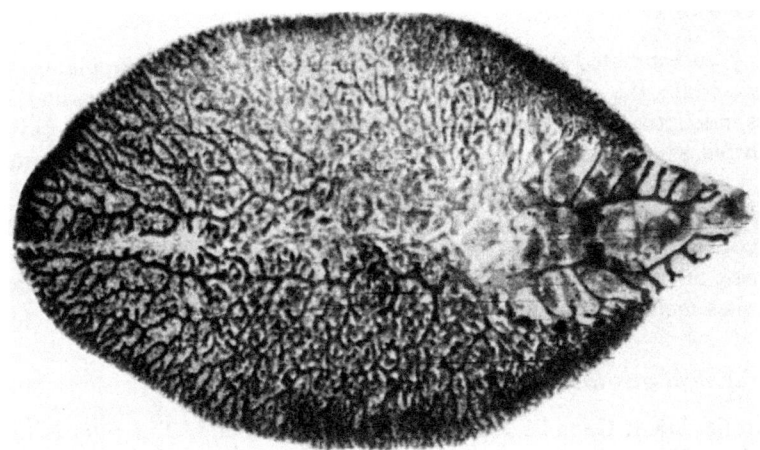

Figure 9.3   The adult liver fluke—an occasional parasite of man

The cercariae of the fluke encyst on any vegetation growing in damp places and thus they may be present on watercress or other aquatic plants which are consumed by man. In this way human infections are set up, and have been reported from Germany, Cuba, Argentina, Russia and the UK.

The symptoms and signs are those of dyspepsia, followed by the sudden onset of high fever, accompanied by abdominal pain which is sometimes acute. The pain lasts for some hours, at first generalized but later becoming localized in the right hypochondrium. The liver becomes palpable and an eosinophilia is found. A latent period then follows in which severe symptoms subside but relapses can occur in which acute symptoms are observed. A third, obstructive phase, can result from obstruction of the bile ducts by flukes or the calculi which accompany them.

Treatment and prevention

Treatment with emetine is usually effective. It seems likely that some of the active, non-toxic fasciolicides recently developed for use in veterinary medicine might be successfully applied although these are not registered for use in man so no proper guidance on their usage is available. Chapter 6 gives further details of treatment.

Prevention for the individual is almost impossible except by eliminating watercress and similar plants from the diet. Various treatments such as hot water which might be expected to kill the cysts are not satisfactory since they also damage the watercress. The best safeguard is to buy watercress from a reputable grower whose establishment and water supply is segregated from farm animals from which contamination could occur.

Echinococcus granulosus

This parasite occurs worldwide and a study of the biological and morphological characteristics of specimens collected in various parts of the world has led some authors to distinguish four subspecies. These are: (a) *E. granulosus granulosus* found in dogs, sheep and other domestic animals; (b) *E. granulosus borealis* found in timber wolves, moose and other cervids indigenous to North America; (c) *E. granulosus canadensis* found in dogs and reindeer; and (d) *E. granulosus equinus* found in dogs and horses. Other authorities consider that a separate subspecies rank for some of these is unjustified and that they are better considered as 'strains' or 'forms'. The definitive host is the dog or other canidae and various mammals serve as an intermediate host as indicated above. Man may be an alternative intermediate host. Infection takes place by the ingestion of eggs of the tapeworm passed in the faeces of dogs harbouring *E. granulosus*. Eggs swallowed by the human host hatch in the intestine and the released oncospheres pass via the portal system to the liver where they develop to hydatid cysts (Figure 9.4). The on-

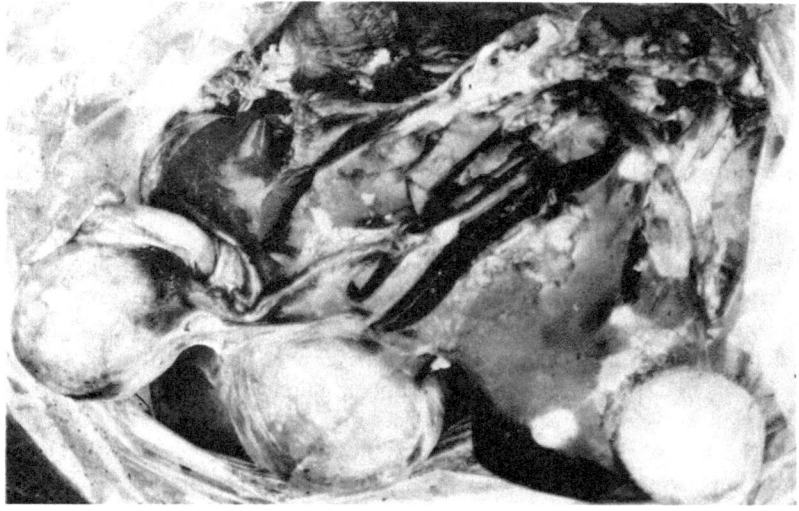

Figure 9.4 Hydatid cysts attached to the liver of a horse

cospheres may pass to other organs such as the lungs, or more rarely to the long bones or the central nervous system where they also develop into cysts. The cyst becomes a large vesicle and scolices bud off from the germinal epithelium of the cyst. If such a cyst is eaten by a dog the scolices develop into tapeworms in its small intestine and so complete the cycle. The tapeworm eggs are more often ingested by sheep, cattle or horses, and it is these species which perpetuate the parasite.

Geographical distribution

Although hydatidosis is of worldwide occurrence, major centres of the disease have been identified in South America, the Mediterranean littoral, South Africa, the Near and Middle East and in parts of North America. Minor centres of hydatidosis are found in many parts of most continents and the disease causes considerable economic loss in farm animals as well as much human illness. In England and Wales there are approximately 10 deaths a year attributable to hydatidosis and one in Scotland. The number of new clinical cases per year in Great Britain averages ten.

Control

The WHO/FAO report on Zoonoses summarized the basic measures for the control of hydatidosis as follows:

1. Eradication of canine infection.
2. Control and elimination of stray dogs.
3. Reduction of populations of wild canidae.
4. The prevention of the reinfection of dogs by the proper disposal of infected organs at slaughterhouses and knackeries.

Not all these methods are applicable to every country. Measure 3, for example, will not be appropriate in many regions. All countries which have a hydatidosis problem implement these measures with varying degrees of diligence and consequently with varying success. In Iceland it has been possible to eradicate the condition completely. In the 19th century the incidence of hydatidosis in Iceland was very high; several factors were responsible for this: the dog population was high (about 15–20 000 compared to a human population of 70 000), housing was poor, and dogs lived in close proximity to their owners (so increasing the chances of infection). One in every four or five persons thus became infected. In 1863 an educational campaign explained the nature of the disease and how to control it. A tax was imposed on the keeping of all dogs except those essential for farm use, but so many were judged 'essential' that the tax was ineffective. Accordingly, in 1890, a tax was imposed on all dogs and the feeding of raw offal to them was forbidden. It became mandatory to burn or bury cysts and a requirement to treat each dog with an anthelminthic annually was enforced. These measures were important in reducing the incidence of hydatid disease, although other factors were equally important. A change took place in the dietary habits of the population: lamb was consumed in preference to mutton from old sheep, thus helping to break the life cycle of the parasite. General improvements in hygiene, housing and the prevention of close contact between the human and dog populations also played a part. Autopsies performed in Reykjavik now only reveal hydatid cysts in persons sufficiently old to have acquired infection before the control measures became effective, thus the disease has now been eliminated from Iceland. In New Zealand similar legislation to control hydatid disease has been in force since 1959. It has reduced the incidence of hydatid disease to a low level, but has not yet succeeded in completely eradicating the disease.

For many years the only satisfactory treatment for *E. granulosus* in dogs was arecoline hydrobromide and this is still used in some countries to diagnose the disease in dogs. After a dose of arecoline the dog purges and any tapeworms present can be recovered from the faeces. More recently bunamidine has been introduced to remove *E. granulosus* in dogs and it is much safer than arecoline. The latest taeniacide for dogs is praziquantel which is highly effective against *E. granulosus* and will be a useful additional aid in the control of hydatid disease.

In summary, control of hydatid disease is achieved by breaking the life cycle. This may be done by eliminating established tapeworm infections in dogs by anthelminthic therapy and by the control of infected offal at the point of slaughter. Infected offal should ideally be destroyed, but if fed to dogs should first be sterilized by boiling.

References for further reading

Gibson, T. E. (1967). Parasitic zoonoses of the food animals in Great Britain. In: Pool, W. A. (ed.) *Veterinary Annual*, 8th year, p. 123

Gould, S. E. (1970). *Trichinosis in Man and Animals*. (Springfield, Illinois: Charles C. Thomas)

Pawlowski, S. and Schultz, M. (1972). Taeniasis and Cysticercosis (*Taenia saginata*). In: Dawes, B. (ed.) *Adv. Parasitol.*, **10**, 269

Ranson, B. H. (1914). The destruction of the vitality of *Cysticercus bovis* by freezing. *J. Parasitol.*, **1**, 5

Report. (1960). Joint WHO/FAO Expert Committee on Zoonoses. Second Report WHO Technical Report Series No. 169

Silverman, P. H. (1955). Bovine cysticerosis in Great Britain from July 1950 to December 1955 with some notes on meat inspection and the incidence of *Taenia saginata* in man. *Ann. Trop. Med. Parasitol.*, **49**, 429

Silverman, P. H. and Griffiths, R. B. (1955). A review of methods of sewage disposal in Great Britain with special reference to the epizootiology of *Cysticercus bovis*. *Ann. Trop. Med. Parasitol.*, **49**, 436

Index